The Little B
Nephrology and
Hypertension

Series Editor: Daniel K. Onion

Charles N. Jacobs, MD
MaineGeneral Medical Center
Division of Nephrology
Waterville, ME
Adjunct Professor of Community and Family Medicine
Dartmouth College Medical School

Dmitry Opolinsky, DO
MaineGeneral Medical Center
Division of Nephrology
Waterville, ME

John Peters, MD
813-332-3554

JONES AND BARTLETT PUBLISHERS
Sudbury, Massachusetts
BOSTON   TORONTO   LONDON   SINGAPORE

World Headquarters

Jones and Bartlett Publishers
40 Tall Pine Drive
Sudbury, MA 01776
978-443-5000
info@jbpub.com
www.jbpub.com

Jones and Bartlett Publishers
Canada
6339 Ormindale Way
Mississauga, Ontario L5V 1J2
CANADA

Jones and Bartlett Publishers
International
Barb House, Barb Mews
London W6 7PA
UK

Jones and Bartlett's books and products are available through most bookstores and online booksellers. To contact Jones and Bartlett Publishers directly, call 800-832-0034, fax 978-443-8000, or visit our website, www.jbpub.com.

Substantial discounts on bulk quantities of Jones and Bartlett's publications are available to corporations, professional associations, and other qualified organizations. For details and specific discount information, contact the special sales department at Jones and Bartlett via the above contact information or send an email to specialsales@jbpub.com.

The authors, editor, and publisher have made every effort to provide accurate information. However, they are not responsible for errors, omissions, or for any outcomes related to the use of the contents of this book and take no responsibility for the use of the products and procedures described. Treatments and side effects described in this book may not be applicable to all people; likewise, some people may require a dose or experience a side effect that is not described herein. Drugs and medical devices are discussed that may have limited availability controlled by the Food and Drug Administration (FDA) for use only in a research study or clinical trial. Research, clinical practice, and government regulations often change the accepted standard in this field. When consideration is being given to use of any drug in the clinical setting, the health care provider or reader is responsible for determining FDA status of the drug, reading the package insert, and reviewing prescribing information for the most up-to-date recommendations on dose, precautions, and contraindications, and determining the appropriate usage for the product. This is especially important in the case of drugs that are new or seldom used.

Library of Congress Cataloging-in-Publication Data

Jacobs, Charles N.
    Little black book of nephrology and hypertension / Charles N. Jacobs and Dmitry Opolinsky.
            p. ; cm. — (Little black book series)
Includes index.
    ISBN-13: 978-0-7637-5297-2
    ISBN-10: 0-7637-5297-5
    1. Nephrology—Handbooks, manuals, etc. 2. Hypertension—Handbooks, manuals,
etc. I. Opolinsky, Dmitry. II. Title. III. Series.
    [DNLM: 1. Kidney Diseases—diagnosis—Handbooks. 2. Hypertension—diagnosis—Handbooks. 3. Hypertension—therapy—Handbooks. 4. Kidney Diseases—therapy—Handbooks. WJ 39 J17L 2009]
    RC902.J33 2009
    616.6'1—dc22
            2008011542

6048

Production Credits

Executive Publisher: Christopher Davis
Senior Acquisition Editor: Nancy Anastasi Duffy
Associate Editor: Kathy Richardson
Associate Production Editor: Mike Boblitt
Associate Marketing Manager: Ilana Goddess
Manufacturing Buyer: Therese Connell

Cover Design: Kristin E. Ohlin
Composition: Publishers' Design and Production Services, Inc.
Cover Image: © Photos.com
Printing and Binding: Malloy, Inc.
Cover Printing: Malloy, Inc.

Printed in the United States of America

12   11   10   09   08   10   9   8   7   6   5   4   3   2   1

Contents

Chapter 4 Glomerular Diseases 109

Chapter 5 Inherited Kidney Diseases 163

Chapter 11 Kidney Transplantation   295

Notice

We have made every attempt to summarize, accurately and concisely, a multitude of references. However the reader is reminded that times and medical knowledge change, transcription or understanding error is always possible, and crucial details are omitted whenever such a comprehensive distillation as this is attempted in limited space. And the primary purpose of this compilation is to cite literature on various sides of controversial issues; knowing where "truth" lies is usually difficult. This book is not intended to be comprehensive as the preface explains. We cannot, therefore, guarantee that every bit of information is absolutely accurate or complete. The reader should affirm that cited recommendations are still reasonable, by reading the original articles and checking other sources including local consultants as well as recent literature before applying them.

Preface

Everything should be made as simple as possible, but not one bit simpler.

Albert Einstein

In this book, the reader will find an overview of the entire field of nephrology and hypertension. We are grateful to Dan Onion for providing us with a format that allows us to discuss common nephrologic conditions in a concise and structured manner.

We have aimed to describe clearly the well-understood principles of everyday nephrology practice in the areas of chronic kidney disease, acute kidney injury, glomerular disease, hypertension, dialysis, and transplantation. In the field of nephrology, recognizable patterns of disease presentations are often easy to confuse with actual treatable conditions. Whenever possible, care was taken to differentiate between patterns of disease that have a differential diagnosis and individual conditions. This book includes many references that will allow the reader to obtain an in-depth understanding of relevant concepts and controversies. It is our hope that this book will serve the reader as a clear and simple guide to today's clinical practice of nephrology.

Charles N. Jacobs
Dmitry Opolinsky

Text Abbreviations

A$_2$	Aortic (first) component of S$_2$	ADPKD	Autosomal Dominant Polycystic Kidney Disease
AA	Alcoholics Anonymous	AED	Automated external defibrillator
AAMI	Association for the Advancement of Medical Instrumentation	AF	Atrial fibrillation
		AFB	Acid-fast bacillus
ab	Antibodies	Afib	Atrial fibrillation
ABGs	Arterial blood gases	Aflut	Atrial flutter
ac	Before meals	AFP	Alpha fetoprotein
AC	Anticoagulate	ag	Antigen
ACE	Angiotensin-converting enzyme	AG	Anion gap
		AGN	Acute glomerular nephritis
ACEI	ACE inhibitor		
Ach	Acetylcholine	AI	Aortic insufficiency
ACLS	Advanced cardiac life support	AIN	Acute interstitial nephritis
ACOG	American College of Obstetrics and Gynecology	aka	Also known as
		AKI	Acute kidney injury
		Al	Aluminum
ACTH	Adrenocorticotropic hormone	ALA	α-Levulinic acid
		ALL	Acute lymphocytic leukemia
AD	Right ear		
ADH	Antidiuretic hormone	ALS	Amyotrophic lateral sclerosis
ADHD	Attention deficit hyperactivity disorder	ALT	SGPT; alanine transferase
ADLs	Activities of daily living	AMI	Anterior myocardial infarction

AML	Acute myelogenous leukemia	AST	SGOT; aspartate transferase
AMR	Antibody mediated (humoral) rejection	asx	Asymptomatic
		atm	Atmospheres
ANA	Antinuclear antibody	ATN	Acute tubular necrosis
ANCA	Antineutrophil cyto-plasmic autoantibodies	AU	Both ears
		AV	Arteriovenous; atrial-ventricular
AODM	Adult-onset diabetes mellitus		
		AVF	arteriovenous fistula
AP	Anterior-posterior	avg	Average
APAS	Antiphospholipid antibody syndrome	AVG	Arteriovenous graft
		AVM	Ateriovenous malformation
APLA	Antiphospholipid antibodies		
AR	Aldose reductase	Ba	Barium
ARA	Angiotensin receptor antagonist	bact	Bacteriology
		BAL	British anti-Lewisite
ARB	Angiotensin receptor blocker	bc	Birth control
		BCG	Bacille Calmette-Guérin
ARDS	Adult respiratory distress syndrome		
		BCLS	Basic cardiac life support
ARPKD	Autosomal recessive polycystic kidney disease		
		bcp's	Birth control pills
		BE	Barium enema
AS	Aortic stenosis; left ear	bid	Twice a day
ASA	Aspirin	BiPAP	Bi (2)-positive airway pressures
asap	As soon as possible		
ASCVD	Arteriosclerotic cardio-vascular disease	biw	Twice a week
		BJ	Bence-Jones
ASD	Atrial septal defect	bm	Bowel movement
ASHD	Arteriosclerotic heart disease	BM	Basement membrane
		BMI	Body mass index
ASLO	Antistreptolysin O titer	BP	Blood pressure
		BPH	Benign prostatic hypertrophy
ASO	Antistreptolysin O titer		
		BS	Blood sugar
		BSE	Breast self-exam

BSOO	Bilateral salpingo-oophorectomy	CIS	Carcinoma in situ
		CKD	Chronic kidney disease
BUN	Blood urea nitrogen	Cl	Chloride
bx	Biopsy	CLIA	Clinical Laboratory Improvement Amendments
C'	Complement		
Ca	Calcium; cancer	CLL	Chronic lymphocytic leukemia
CABG	Coronary artery bypass graft	CMF	Cytoxan, methotrexate, 5-FU
CAD	Coronary artery disease		
cAMP	Cyclic AMP	CML	Chronic myelocytic leukemia
CAN	Chronic allograft nephropathy		
		cmplc	Complications
CAPD	Continuous ambulatory peritoneal dialysis	CMV	Cytomegalovirus
		CN	Cranial nerve; cyanide
cath	Catheterization	CNS	Central nervous system
CBC	Complete blood count	c/o	Complaining of
CBCD	Complete blood count and differential	CO	Cardiac output
		col	Colonies
cc	Cubic centimeter	COLA	Cystine, ornithine, lysine, and arginine
CCPD	Continuous cycling peritoneal dialysis		
		COPD	Chronic obstructive lung disease
CEA	Carcinoembryonic antigen		
		cp	Cerebellar-pontine
cf	Compare	CP	Cerebral palsy
CF	Complement fixation antibodies; cystic fibrosis	CPAP	Continuous positive airway pressure
		CPC	Clinical/pathologic conference
CHD	Congenital heart disease		
		CPG	Coproporphyrinogen
chem	Chemistries	CPK	Creatine phophokinase
chemoRx	Chemotherapy	CPR	Cardiopulmonary resuscitation
CHF	Congestive heart failure		
		cps	Cycles per second
CI	Cardiac index	Cr	Creatinine
CIN	Chronic interstitial nephritis	CREST	Calcinosis, Raynaud's, esophageal

	reflux, sclerodactyly, telangiectasias	D + E	Dilatation and evacuation (suction)
CRH	Corticotropin-releasing hormone	DES	Diethyl stilbesterol
crit	Hematocrit	DEXA	Dual Energy X-Ray Absorptiometry
CRP	C reactive protein	DHS	Delayed hypersensitivity
crs	Course		
c + s	Culture and sensitivity	DI	Diabetes insipidus
C/S	Cesarean section	dias	Diastolic
CSF	Cerebrospinal fluid	DIC	Disseminated intravascular coagulation
CT	Computerized tomography		
		dig	Digoxin
CTA	Computed tomography angiogram	dip	Distal interphalangeal joint
Cu	Copper	DJD	Degenerative joint disease
CVA	Cerebrovascular accident		
		DKA	Diabetic ketoacidosis
CVP	Central venous pressure	DM	Diabetes mellitus
		DMSA	Dimercaptosuccinic acid
CVVH	Continuous veno-venous hemofiltration		
		DNA	Deoxyribonucleic acid
CVVHD	Continuous veno-venous hemodialysis	d/o	Disorder
		DOE	Dyspnea on exertion
CVVHDF	Continuous veno-venous hemodiafiltration	D/P	Dialysate-to-plasma
		DPG	Diphosphoglycerate
		DPI	Dry powder inhaler
CXR	Chest Xray	DPN	Diphosphopyridine nucleotide
d	Day(s)	DPNH	Reduced DPN
DAT	Dementia, Alzheimer's type	DPT	Diphtheria, pertussus, tetanus vaccine
dB	Decibel	DRIL	Distal revascularization with interval ligation
dL	Deciliter		
DBCT	Double-blind controlled trial	DS	Double strength
		dT	Diphtheria tetanus adult vaccine
D + C	Dilatation and curettage		

DTaP	Diphtheria, tetanus, acellular pertussis vaccine	ESR	Erythrocyte sedimentation rate
DTRs	Deep tendon reflexes	ESRD	End-stage renal disease
DTs	Delirium tremens	et	Endotracheal
DU	Duodenal ulcer	et al	And others
DVT	Deep venous thrombosis	etc	And so forth
dx	Diagnosis or diagnostic	ETOH	Ethanol
		ETT	Exercise tolerance test
		F	Female; Fahrenheit
EACA	ε-Aminocaproic acid	FA	Fluorescent antibody; folic acid
EBV	Epstein-Barr virus		
ECM	Erythema chronicum marginatum	FBS	Fasting blood sugar
		Fe	Iron
EF	Ejection fraction	FEV_1	Forced expiratory vital capacity in 1 second
eg	For example		
EGD	Esophagogastro-duodenoscopy	FFA	Free fatty acids
		FFP	Fresh frozen plasma
EKG	Electrocardiogram	FIGLU	Formiminoglutamic acid
ELISA	Enzyme-linked immu-nosorbent assay		
		fl	Femtoliter
E/M	Erythroid/myeloid	FMF	Familial Mediterrra-nean fever
EM	Electron microscopy		
EMG	Electromyogram	freq	Frequency
EMT	Emergency Medical Technician	FSGS	Focal segmental glomerulosclerosis
Endo	Endoscopy	FSH	Follicle-stimulating hormone
Epidem	Epidemiology		
ER	Estrogen receptors; emergency room	FTA	Fluorescent treponemal antibody
ERCP	Endoscopic retro-grade cholangio-pancreatography	FTT	Failure to thrive
		f/u	Follow up
		FUO	Fever of unknown origin
ERT	Estrogen replacement therapy	FVC	Forced vital capacity
ESA	Erythropoietic stimu-lating agents	fx	Fracture

g	Gauge	H & E	Hematoxylin and eosin
GABA	γ-Aminobutyric acid	hem	Hematology
gc	Gonorrhea	hep	Hepatitis
GE	Gastroesophageal	H. flu	*Hemophilus influenzae*
GFR	Glomerular filtration rate	Hg	Mercury
		hgb	Hemoglobin
GHRH	Growth hormone–releasing hormone	HgbA$_1$C	Hemoglobin A$_1$C level
		HGH	Human growth hormone
gi	Gastrointestinal		
glu	Glucose	5-HIAA	5-Hydroxy indole acedic acid
glut	Glutamine		
gm	Gram	Hib	*Hemophilus influenzae* B vaccine
GN	Glomerulonephritis		
GnRH	Gonadotropin-releasing hormone	his	Histidine
		HIV	Human immunodeficiency virus
GTT	Glucose tolerance test		
gtts	Drops	HLA	Human leukocyte antigens
gu	Genitourinary		
GVHD	Graft-vs-host disease	HMG	Hydroxymethylglutaryl-CoA (coenzyme A)
HAART	Highly active antiretroviral therapy		
		h/o	History of
HAMA	Human anti-mouse antibodies	H&P	History and physical
		hpf	High-power field
HBIG	Hepatitis B immune globulin	HPV	Human papillomavirus
		hr	Hour(s)
HCG	Human chorionic gonadotropin	HRIG	Human rabies immune globulin
HCGrH	HCG-releasing hormone	HRS	Hepatorenal syndrome
		hs	At bedtime
HCl	Hydrochloric acid	HSP	Henoch-Schonlein purpura
HCO$_3$	Bicarbonate		
hct	Hematocrit	HSV	Herpes simplex virus
hemodialysis HD		HT	Hypertension
HDL	High-density lipoprotein	5HT	5-Hydroxytryptophan

HUS	Hemolytic uremic syndrome	IPG	Impedance plethysmography
HVA	Homovanillic acid	IPPB	Intermittent positive pressure breathing
hx	History		
		IPPD	Intermediate purified protein derivative
I or I_2	Iodine		
IADLs	Instrumental activities of daily living	IQ	Intelligence quotient
		ITP	Idiopathic thrombocytopenic purpura
IBD	Inflammatory bowel disease		
		IU	International units
ibid	Same reference as last reference above	IUD	Intrauterine device
		IUGR	Intrauterine growth retardation
ICU	Intensive care unit		
I+D	Incision and drainage	iv	Intravenous
IDDM	Insulin-dependent diabetes mellitus	IVC	Inferior vena cava
		IVP	Intravenous pyleogram
IDPN	intradialytic parenteral nutrition	IWMI	Inferior wall myocardial infarction
ie	In other words		
IEP	Immunoelectrophoresis	J	Joule
IF	Intrinsic factor	JODM	Juvenile-onset diabetes mellitus
IFA	Immunofluorescent antibody		
		JRA	Juvenile rheumatoid arthritis
IgA	Immunoglobulin A		
IgE	Immunoglobulin E	JVD	Jugular venous distention
IgG	Immunoglobulin G		
IgM	Immunoglobulin M	JVP	Jugular venous pressure/pulse
IHSS	Idiopathic hypertrophic subaortic stenosis		
IL-2	Interleukin-2	K	Potassium
im	Intramuscular	KDOQI	Kidney Disease Outcomes Quality Initiative
incr	Increased		
INH	Isoniazid		
INR	International normalized ratio (protimes)	kg	Kilogram
		KOH	Potassium hydroxide
IP	Interphalangeal	KS	Kaposi's sarcoma

KUB	Abdominal X-ray ("kidneys, ureters, bladder")	MAST	Military antishock trousers
		MCD	Minimal change disease
L	Liter; left	mcp	Metacarpal-phalangeal joint
LA	Left atrium; long acting		
LAP	Leukocyte alkaline phosphatase	MD	Muscular dystrophy; physician
LATS	Long-acting thyroid-stimulating protein	MDI	Metered-dose inhaler
		meds	Medications
LBBB	Left bundle branch block	MEN	Multiple endocrine neoplasias
LCCD	Light Chain Deposition Disease	mEq	Millieqivalent
		mets	Metastases
LDH	Lactate dehydrogenase	METs	Metabolic equivalents
LDL	Low-density lipoprotein	MHC	Major histocompatibility complex
LES	Lower esophageal sphincter	mg	Milligram
		Mg	Magnesium
LFTs	Liver function tests	MI	Myocardial infarction; mitral insufficiency
LH	Luteinizing hormone		
LHRH	LH-releasing hormone	MIBG	I-123 metaiodobenzyl-guanidine
LMW	Low molecular weight		
LP	Lumbar puncture	MIC	Minimum inhibitory concentration
LS	Lumbosacral		
LV	Left ventricle	MID	Multi-infarct dementia
LVH	Left ventricular hypertrophy	min	Minute(s)
		MM	Multiple myeloma
lytes	Electrolytes	MMF	Mycophenolate mofetil
		MMR	Measles, mumps, rubella
m	Meter(s)		
M	Male	MN	Membranous Nephropathy
MAI	*Mycobacterium avium intracellulare*		
		mOsm	Milliosmole(s)
MAO	Monamine oxidase	mp	Metocarpal phalangeal
MAP	Mean arterial pressure	MPGN	Membranoproliferative glomerulonephritis

6MP	6-Mercaptopurine	NICU	Newborn intensive care unit
MR	Mitral regurgitation		
MRA	Magnetic resonance angiography	NIDDM	Non-insulin-dependent diabetes mellitus
MRFIT	Multiple risk factor intervention trial	nl	Normal
		nL	Nanoliter(s)
MRI	Magnetic resonance imaging	nm	Nanometer(s)
		NMRI	Nuclear magnetic resonance imaging
MRSA	Methicillin-resistant *Staphylococcus aureus*	NMS	Neuroleptic malignant syndrome
MS	Multiple sclerosis; mitral stenosis	NNH	Number needed to harm
MSH	Melanocyte-stimulating hormone	NNT	Number needed to treat
MTOR	Mammalian target of rapamycin	NNT-5	NNT over 5 years
mtx	Methotrexate	noninv	Noninvasive
μ	Micron(s)	NPH	Normal-pressure hydrocephalus
μgm	Microgram(s)		
Multip	Multiparous patient	npo	Nothing by mouth
		NS	Normal saline
Na	Sodium	NSAID	Nonsteroidal anti-inflammatory drug
NAD	Nicotinamide adenine dinucleotide	NSR	Normal sinus rhythm
NADH	Reduced form of NAD	NST	Nonstress test
NCI	National Cancer Institute	Nullip	Nulliparous patient
		NV+D	Nausea, vomiting, and diarrhea
ncnc	Normochromic normocytic		
NCV	Nerve conduction velocities	O₂	Oxygen
		OB	Obstetrics
neb	Nebulizer	OCD	Obsessive-compulsive disorder
neg	Negative		
NG	Nasogastric	OD	Overdose; right eye
NH	Nursing home	OGTT	Oral glucose tolerance test
NH₃	Ammonia		
		OH	Hydroxy-

OM	Otitis media	PCTA	Percutaneous translu-minal angioplasty
op	Operative; outpatient		
O+P	Ova and parasites	PCWP	Pulmonary capillary wedge pressure
OPD	Outpatient department		
OPV	Oral polio vaccine	PD	Peritoneal dialysis
OS	Left eye	PDA	Patent ductus arteriosus
osm	Osmole(s)		
OTC	Over the counter	PEG	Percutaneous endo-scopic gastrostomy
OU	Both eyes		
oz	Ounce	PEP	Protein electrophoresis
		PERRLA	Pupils equal round reactive to light and accommodation
P	Pulse		
P_2	Pulmonary (second) component of S_2		
		PET	Pritoneal equilibration test
PA	Pernicious anemia; pulmonary artery		
		PFTs	Pulmonary function tests
PABA	Paraminobenzoic acid		
PAC	Premature atrial contraction	PG	Prostaglandin
		PHLA	Post-heparin lipolytic activity
PAF	Paroxysmal atrial fibrillation		
		PI	Pulmonic insufficiency
PAN	Polyarteritis nodosa	PID	Pelvic inflammatory disease
Pap	Papanicolaou		
PAP	Pulmonary artery pressure	PIH	Pregnancy-induced hypertension
par	Parenteral	pip	Proximal interphalan-geal joint
PAS	p-Amino salicylic acid		
PAT	Paroxysmal atrial tachycardia	PMI	Point of maximal impulse of heart
pathophys	Pathophysiology	PML	Progressive multifocal leukoencephalopathy
Pb	Lead		
PBG	Porphobilinogen	PMNLs	Polymorphonuclear leukocytes
pc	After meals		
PCP	*Pneumocystis carinii* pneumonia	PMR	Polymyalgia rheumatica
PCR	Polymerase chain reaction	PND	Paroxysmal nocturnal dyspnea

PNH	Paroxysmal hemoglobinuria	PTRA	Percutaneous transmural renal angiography
po	By mouth	PTT	Partial thromboplastin time
PO4	Phosphate		
polys	Polymorphonuclear leukocytes	PUD	Peptic ulcer disease
		PUVA	Psoralen + UVA light
pos	Positive	PVC	Premature ventricular tachycardia
post-op	Postoperative		
PP	Protoporphyrin		
ppd	Pack per day	q	Every
PPD	Tuberculin skin test	qd	Daily
PPG	Protoporphyrinogen	qid	4 times a day
pr	By rectum	qod	Every other day
PRA	Panel reactive antibody	qow	Every other week
pRBBB	Partial right bundle branch block	qt	Quart
pre-op	Pre-operative	R	Right; respirations
prep	Preparation	RA	Rheumatoid arthritis
primip	Primiparous patient	RAIU	Radioactive iodine uptake
prn	As needed		
PROM	Premature rupture of membranes	RAST	Radioallergosorbent test
PS	Pulmonic stenosis	RBBB	Right bundle branch block
PSA	Prostate-specific antigen		
		rbc	Red blood cell
PSVT	Paroxysmal supraventricular tachycardia	RCT	Randomized controlled trial
pt(s)	Patient(s)	RDBCT	Randomized double-blind trial
PT	Protime		
PTDM	Post-transplant diabetes mellitus	RDS	Respiratory distress syndrome
PTFE	Polytetrafluoroethylene	re	About
PTH	Parathyroid hormone	rehab	Rehabilitation
PTLD	Post-transplant lymphoproliferative disorder	REM	Rapid eye movement
		RES	Reticuloendothelial system
		retic	Reticulocyte(s)

Rh	Rhesus factor	Sb	Antimony
RHD	Rheumatic heart disease	SBE	Subacute bacterial endocarditis
RIA	Radioimmunoassay	SBP	Spontaneous bacterial peritonitis
RIBA	Radio-immunoblot assay	sc	Subcutaneous
RKF	Residual kidney function	SCUF	Slow continuous ultrafiltration
RMSF	Rocky Mountain spotted fever	SD	Standard deviation
ROM	Range of motion	sens	Sensitivity
ROS	Review of systems	SER	Smooth endoplasmic reticulum
RNA	Ribonucleic acid	serol	Serology
RNP	Ribonucleoprotein	SGA	Small for gestational age
r/o	Rule out	si	Sign(s)
RPGN	Rapidly progressive glomerulonephritis	SI	Sacroiliac
RSV	Respiratory syncytial virus	SIADH	Syndrome of inappropriate ADH
RTA	Renal tubular acidosis	SIDS	Sudden infant death syndrome
RRT	Renal replacement therapy	SKSD	Streptokinase, streptodornase
rv	Review	sl	Sublingual
RV	Right ventricle	SLE	Systemic lupus erythematosus
RVH	Right ventricular hypertrophy	SLEDD	Slow low efficiency daily dialysis
rx	Treatment	SNF	Skilled nursing facility
S_1	First heart sound	soln	Solution
S_2	Second heart sound	s/p	Status post
S_3	Third heart sound, gallop	specif	Specificity
S_4	Fourth heart sound, gallop	SPEP	Serum protein electrophoresis
SAB	Spontaneous abortion	SR	Slow release
SAH	Subarachnoid hemorrhage	SRS	Slow-reacting substance

SS	Sickle cell disease	TENS	Transcutaneous electrical nerve stimulation
SSI	Sliding-scale insulin		
SSKI	Saturated solution of potassium iodide	tfx	Transfusion
		THC	Tetrahydro-cannabinol
SSRI	Selective serotonin reuptake inhibitor	TI	Tricuspid insufficiency
		TIA	Transient ischemic attack
SSS	Sick sinus syndrome		
staph	*Staphylococcus*	TIBC	Total iron-binding capacity
STD	Sexually transmitted disease		
		tid	3 times a day
strep	*Streptococcus*	TIPS	Transjugular intrahepatic portosystemic shunt
STS	Serologic test for syphilis		
SVC	Superior vena cava	tiw	Three times a week
SVT	Supraventricular tachycardia	TMA	Thrombotic microangiopathy
sx	Symptom(s)	TTKG	Transtubular potassium gradient
T°	Fever/temperature	Tm	Trimethoprim
T_3	Triiodothyronine	TM	Tympanic membrane
T_4	Thyroxin	Tm/S	Trimethoprim/sulfa
T+A	Tonsillectomy and adenoidectomy	TNF	Tumor necrosis factor
		TNG	Nitroglycerine
TA	Temporal arteritis	TNM	Tumor, nodes, metastases
tab	Tablet		
TAH	Total abdominal hysterectomy	TPA	Tissue plasminogen activator
tbc	Tuberculosis	TPN	Total parental nutrition
TBG	Thyroid-binding globulin		
		TPNH	Triphosphopyridine reduced
TCAs	Tricyclic antidepressants	TRH	Thyroid-releasing hormone
tcn	Tetracycline		
Td	Tetanus/diphtheria, adult type	TS	Tricuspid stenosis
		TSAT	Transferrin saturation
TEE	Transesophageal echocardiogram	TSH	Thyroid-stimulating hormone

tsp	Teaspoon(s)	VMA	Vanillymandelic acid
TTP	Thrombotic thrombo-cytopenic purpura	vol	Volume
		V/Q	Ventilation/perfusion
TURP	Transurethral resection of prostate	vs	versus
		VSD	Ventricular septal defect
U	Unit(s)	VT or Vtach	Ventricular tachycardia
UA	Urinalysis	VWF	von Willebrand factor
UBO	Unidentified bright object	V-ZIG	Varicella-zoster immune globulin
UGI	Upper gastrointestinal		
UGIS	Upper gastrointestinal series	w	With
		wbc	White blood cells; white blood count
URI	Upper respiratory illness	WHO	World Health Organization
URR	Urea reduction ratio		
U.S.	United States	wk	Week(s)
US	Ultrasound	WNL	Within normal limits
USPTF	U.S. Preventive Task Force	WPW	Wolff-Parkinson-White syndrome (short PR interval)
UTI	Urinary tract infection		
UUB	Urine urobilinogen	W/s	Watt/second
UV	Ultraviolet	w/u	Work up
UVA	Ultraviolet A		
UVB	Ultraviolet B	xmatch	Cross-match
vag	Vaginally	yr	Year(s)
val	Valine		
VCUG	Vesico-urethrogram	ZE	Zollinger-Ellison syndrome
VDRL	Serologic test for syphilis (Venereal Disease Research Lab)		
		Zn	Zinc
		>	More than
VF or Vfib	Ventricular fibrillation	>>	Much more than
VIP	Vasoactive intestinal peptide	<	less than
		<<	Much less than
VLDL	Very-low-density lipoprotein	$\varnothing$	Leads to (eg, in a chemical reaction)

Journal Abbreviations

Adolesc Med Clin	Adolescent Medicine Clinics of North America
Adv Perit Dial	Advances in Peritoneal Dialysis
Am Fam Physician	American Family Physician
Am J Roentgenol	American Journal of Roentgenology
Am J Cardiol	American Journal of Cardiology
Am J Epidemiol	American Journal of Epidemiology
Am J Emerg Med	American Journal of Emergency Medicine
Am J Hematol	American Journal of Hematology
Am J Kidney Dis	American Journal of Kidney Disease
Am J Med	American Journal of Medicine
Am J Med Sci	American Journal of Medical Science
Am J Nephrol	American Journal of Nephrology
Am J Transplant	American Journal of Transplantation
Am Heart J	American Heart Journal
Ann Intern Med	Annals of Internal Medicine
Ann Oncol	Annals of Oncology
Ann Pharmacother	Annals of Pharmacotherapy
Annu Rev Med	Annual Review of Medicine
Arch Intern Med	Archives of Internal Medicine
Arthritis Rheum	Arthritis and Rheumatism
Aust Fam Physician	Australian Family Physician
Best Pract Res Clin Endocrinol Metab	Best Practice & Research Clinical Endocrinology & Metabolism
Blood Press Monit	Blood Pressure Monitoring
Blood Purif	Blood Purification
Blood Rev	Blood Reviews
BMC Nephrol	BMC Nephrology

Br Med J	British Medical Journal
Br J Haematol	British Journal of Haematology
Cardiol Rev	Cardiology Reviews
Clin Chest Med	Clinics in Chest Medicine
Clin J Am Soc Nephrol	Clinical Journal of the American Society of Nephrology
Clin J Sport Med	Clinical Journal of Sports Medicine
Clin Liver Dis	Clinical Liver Disease
Clin Nephrol	Clinical Nephrology
Clin Transpl	Clinical Transplantation
Clin Sci	Clinical Science
CMAJ	Canadian Medical Association Journal
Cochrane Database Syst Rev	Cochrane Database of Systematic Reviews
Crit Care Med	Critical Care Medicine
Curr Hypertens Rep	Current Hypertension Reviews
Curr Opin Crit Care	Current Opinion in Critical Care
Curr Opin Pediatr	Current Opinion in Pediatrics
Drug Alcohol Rev	Drug and Alcohol Review
Drug Saf	Drug Safety
Emerg Med Clin North Am	Emergency Medicine Clinics of North America
Emerg Med J	Emergency Medicine Journal
Eur J Vasc Endovasc Surg	European Journal of Vascular and Endovascular Surgery
Endocrinol Metab Clin North Am	Endocrinology and Metabolism Clinics of North America
Gastrointest Endosc	Gastrointestinal Endoscopy
Hematol Oncol Clin North Am	Hematology and Oncology Clinics of North America

Hemodial Int	Hemodialysis International
Hypertens Res	Hypertension Research
Int J Cancer	International Journal of Cancer
Intensive Care Med	Intensive Care Medicine
JAMA	Journal of the American Medical Association
J Am Coll Cardiol	Journal of the American College of Cardiology
J Am Geriatr Soc	Journal American Geriatric Society
J Am Soc Nephrol	Journal American Society of Nephrology
J Clin Endocrinol Metab	Journal of Clinical Endocrinology and Metabolism
J Clin Hypertens	Journal of Clinical Hypertension
J Gastroenterol Hepatol	Journal of Gastroenterology and Hepatology
J Clin Invest	Journal of Clinical Investigation
J Gen Intern Med	Journal of General Internal Medicine
J Fam Pract	Journal of Family Practice
J Hypertens	Journal of Hypertension
J Nephrol	Journal of Nephrology
J Pediatr	Journal of Pediatrics
J Physiol	Journal of Physiology
J Paediatr Child Health	Journal of the Paediatrics and Child Health
J Toxicol Clin Toxicol	Journal of Toxicology. Clinical Toxicology
J Urol	Journal of Urology
J Vasc Surg	Journal of Vascular Surgery
J Urol	Journal of Urology
Kidney Int	Kidney International
Mayo Clin Proc	Mayo Clinic Proceedings
Magnes Res	Magnesium Research
Med Lett Drugs Ther	The Medical Letter on Drugs and Therapeutics
MMWR	Morbidity and Mortality Weekly Report
Nat Clin Pract Nephrol	Nature Clinical Practice. Nephrology
N Engl J Med	New England Journal of Medicine
Nephrol Dial Transplant	Nephrology Dialysis Transplantation

Obstet Gynecol	Obstetrics and Gynecology
Otolaryngol Head Neck Surg	**Otolaryngology and Head and Neck Surgery**
Pediatr Clin North Am	Pediatric Clinics of North America
Perit Dial Int	Peritoneal Dialysis International
Postgrad Med J	Postgraduate Medical Journal
Prenat Diagn	Prenatal Diagnosis
Ren Fail	Renal Failure
Rev Saude Publica	Revista de Saúde Pública
Scand J Clin Lab Invest	Scandinavian Journal of Laboratory Investigation
Semin Dial	Seminars in Dialysis
Semin Nephrol	Seminars in Nephrology
Semin Oncol	Seminars in Oncology
Semin Vasc Surg	Seminars in Vascular Surgery
Transplant Proc	Proceedings of the Clinical Dialysis and Transplant Forum
Urol Clin North Am	Urology Clinics of North America

Chapter 1

Electrolyte Disorders

1.1 Hyponatremia

Cause: Several clinical scenarios present with hyponatremia. An
evaluation of the patient's volume status and the measured serum
osmolality are used to distinguish among them. Hypoosmolar
hyponatremia is characterized by 3 volume states: hypovolemic,
euvolemic, and edematous. Hyperosmolar hyponatremia is distin-
guished by a normal or elevated serum osmolality.

- *Hypovolemic, hypoosmolar:*
  - Volume contraction due to urinary, gastrointestinal, and/
    or insensible losses with partial repletion by hypotonic
    solutions. Overuse of diuretics and gastroenteritis are some
    clinical situations.
- *Euvolemic, hypoosmolar:*
  - SIADH
    Common medications that induce SIADH are chlorpro-
    pamide, carbamazepine, oxcarbamazepine, cyclophosphamide,
    and SSRI. Pulmonary tumors, infections, and surgery can cause
    SIADH. Neurologic conditions such as stroke and infection
    and even pain can cause SIADH. SIADH can not be reliably
    diagnosed in the setting of heart failure, liver failure, or kidney
    failure.
  - Exogenous administration of ADH, vasopressin
  - Thiazide diuretics (Am J Nephrol 1999;19:4)
  - Cerebral salt wasting

- Hypothyroidism
- Adrenal insufficiency
- Polydipsia
- *Edematous state, hypoosmolar:*
  - Kidney failure
  - Heart failure
  - Liver failure
- *Hyperosmolar:*
  - Hyperglycemia
  - Glycine absorption following transurethral resection of the prostate
  - Mannitol infusion
  - Ethylene glycol ingestion

Note: Hyperlipidemia and dysproteinemia do not cause a factitious lowering of the sodium concentration when measured with modern laboratory equipment using the ion selective electrode.

Epidem: Na < 136 mEq/L has been found to be in 30%–42% of hospitalized patients and Na < 126 mEq/L in 2.6%–6.2%. Often (up to 67% of the time), it develops during the hospital stay. Older age is a risk factor for this abnormality. It is seen in up to 30% of patients hospitalized with cirrhosis and up to 21% of patients hospitalized with severe CHF (Am J Med 2006;119[suppl 1]:7). It develops in a small number of endurance athletes by the end of an event (< 1%) (Clin J Sport Med 2003;13:1). It is more common in women and racers with longer finish times (N Engl J Med 2005;352:15). Risk factors for developing hyponatremia on SSRI include older age, female sex, and concurrent use of diuretics (Ann Pharmacother 2006;40:9).

Pathophys: ADH production is stimulated by ineffective circulating volume and elevated osmolar levels. ADH opens the water channels (aquaporins) in the cortical and medullary collecting tubules allowing for the reabsorption of water from the glomerular filtrate. The hypoosmolar state causes movement of water into the brain cells. When this occurs rapidly, brain swelling can occur. When the state develops slowly, the brain is stimulated to excrete intracellular potassium stores and organic osmoles. This returns the size of the cells toward normal. In situations with decreased effective circulating volume due to hypovolemia, CHF, or cirrhosis, the stimulus for ADH production overrides the stimulus to suppress it from the hypoosmolar state. Patients with kidney failure may be unable to excrete a water load despite a suppressed ADH level. In hyperosmolar hyponatremia, the osmotically active substance in the plasma causes water to move out of cells, which dilutes the sodium concentration. In addition, the hyperosmolar state stimulates thirst and the intake of water, which further reduces the sodium concentration.

Sx: The central nervous system is the target of the syndromes associated with hypoosmolar hyponatremia. Lethargy, muscle cramps, anorexia, confusion, coma, and seizure appear when sodium levels are less than 125 mEq/L. Symptoms are more likely when the condition develops acutely (< 48 hr). Chronic hyponatremia is often asymptomatic.

In hypovolemic hyponatremia, the symptoms of volume depletion predominate: low blood pressure, tachycardia, orthostatic hypotension, poor skin turgor, and dry mucous membranes.

Hyponatremia in edematous states is noted for edema and other signs of extravascular volume overload: pulmonary edema with heart failure, ascites in liver failure, and hypertension in kidney failure.

Since hyperosmolar hyponatremia has a normal or elevated serum osmolality, there are no symptoms directly attributable to the sodium concentration.

Crs: Acute symptomatic hypoosmolar hyponatremia can lead to permanent brain damage and death from the brain swelling.

Cmplc:

- Too rapid correction of chronic hypoosmolar hyponatremia can lead to central pontine myelinolysis. Possible mechanisms include excessive shrinkage of endothelial cells, which disrupts the blood-brain barrier, and cellular death caused by the rapid change in sodium concentration.
- CHF with hyponatremia at presentation predicts higher mortality (Am J Cardiol 2005;96:12A).
- Hyponatremia in cirrhosis is a predictor of poor prognosis (Hepatology 2006;44:6).

Lab: Serum osmolality, urine osmolality; urine Na; uric acid; TSH, cortisol; electrolytes; BUN; creatinine; glucose; urine dipstick (See Table 1.1.)

Table 1.1   Interpretation of Laboratory Findings in Hyponatremia

Condition	Serum Osmolality	Urine Osmolality	Urine Na	Uric Acid	Other
SIADH	< 260 mOsm/L	> 300 mOsm/L	> 40 mEq/L	< 4 mg/dL	
Polydipsia	< 260 mOsm/L	< 100 mOsm/L			Urine specific gravity < 1.003
Hypovolemia (ineffective circulating volume)	< 260 mOsm/L	> 200 mOsm/L (often > 600 mOsm/L)	< 20 mEq/L (except when on diuretics)	Normal or high (> 7 mg/dL)	BUN/Creatinine ratio > 20
Thiazide diuretics	< 260 mOsm/L			> 7 mg/dL	Low K
Hyperosmolar hyponatremia	> 280 mOsm/L				Osmolar gap* > 20

*Osmolar gap = serum osmolality − (2x Na + glucose/180 + BUN/2.8).

Xray: CXR and head CT to look for pulmonary or neurological causes of SIADH

Rx:

- *Hypovolemic hypoosmolar:* Initial treatment with normal saline to replenish volume status is indicated; however, when the patient's volume status is restored, a water diuresis will ensue, which will cause a rapid rise in the serum sodium concentration. At this time, administration of hypotonic solution should be started.
- *Euvolemic hypoosmolar:* Chronic symptomatic hyponatremia presents a therapeutic challenge because too rapid correction is a risk for central pontine myelinolysis. The deficit in sodium from the desired Na concentration (usually 120 mEq/L or 12 mEq/L higher than the presenting value) can be calculated as follows:

$$\text{Na deficit (mEq)} = [\text{desired Na (mEq/L)} - \text{serum Na (mEq/L)}] \times [0.6 \times \text{Wt(kg)}]$$

3% saline contains 513 mEq NaCl/L, and the appropriate quantity should be administered at a rate to raise the serum sodium between 0.5 and 1 mEq/hr. The goal for increase in sodium correction in a 24-hour period should be 12 mEq/L. An alternative approach is to use a combination of normal saline and a loop diuretic. This is especially effective when the urine osmolality can be brought below 400 mOsm/L. Because of ongoing urinary and insensible losses during treatment, frequent monitoring is required. The serum sodium concentration should be checked every 4 hours. Urinary osmolality and urine sodium concentration should be repeated at least daily. If the rate of correction is too rapid, a change to a hypotonic intravenous solution should be made. Acute symptomatic hyponatremia can be corrected more rapidly. The approach to asymptomatic hyponatremia is much different. A water restriction to 1 L daily is indicated. An increase in solute load is encouraged with liberal salt and protein intake in the diet. Removal of any medications that could be responsible and reversal of an underlying cause are also indicated. Clinical trials with several vasopressin V2 receptor antagonists have shown that they can raise the serum sodium in patients with CHF, cirrhosis, and SIADH. Conivaptan (a V1a/V2 vasopressin receptor antagonist) is approved for the treatment of euvolemic hyponatremia. A 20 mg IV loading dose is followed by a continuous infusion at a rate of 20 mg/d for up to 4 days (Med Lett Drugs Ther 2006;48:1237).

- *Edematous state, hypoosmolar:* Patients with edematous states should be treated with fluid restriction and loop diuretics.
- *Hyperosmolar:* In the case of hyperosmolar hyponatremia, the underlying disorder should be corrected. When advanced kidney failure is present, hemodialysis can be used to remove the osmotically active substance.

1.2 Hypernatremia

Cause:

- Decreased water intake: volume depletion with inadequate access to water
- Excess water loss: nephrogenic diabetes insipidus, central diabetes insipidus, loop diuretics, lithium, osmotic diuresis, hypercalcemia, hypokalemia
- Excess salt intake: near drowning in salt water, administration of hypertonic iv solutions, administration of hypertonic oral rehydration solutions in infants

Epidem: 1% of hospitalized patients, up to 30% of elderly patients, admitted from a nursing home (J Am Geriatr Soc 1988;36:213).

Pathophys: The central nervous system is the target of the symptoms. The high serum osmolality causes intracellular volume contraction. This can disrupt neuron function. Rapid and severe volume loss in the cranium can lead to intracranial hemorrhage. If the condition occurs slowly, the neurons adapt to hypertonicity with the uptake of organic osmolytes to defend their volume. This adaptation takes several days to become effective.

Sx: Lethargy, confusion, coma; often associated with signs of volume depletion

Crs: Mortality in the elderly can be higher than 50% and is associated with hypotension on presentation (Am J Emerg Med 1997;15:130).

Cmplc: Intracranial hemorrhage

Lab: Electrolytes, BUN, creatinine, glucose, calcium, urine osmolality, urine Na, urinalysis (See Table 1.2)

Table 1.2   Interpretation of Urinary Findings in Hypernatremia

Condition	Finding
Volume depletion	Urine specific gravity > 1.020 (Urine osmolality > 600 mOsm/L) Urine Na < 10 mEq/L
Osmotic diuresis	Urine specific gravity = 1.010 (Urine osmolality = 300 mOsm/L)
Central or nephrogenic DI, loop diuretics	Urine specific gravity < 1.006 (Urine osmolality < 250 mOsm/L)

Xray: CT scan of head to look for a hypothalamic lesion or intracranial hemorrhage

Rx: Because of the high mortality of hypernatremia associated with volume depletion, these patients must be adequately fluid resuscitated. The initial intravenous fluids should be normal saline, and when the vital signs are stabilized, a change to 1/2 normal saline should be made.

For euvolemic or volume overloaded patients, the free water deficit should be calculated:

$$\text{Free water deficit (L)} = \text{wt (kg)} \times 0.6 \left([\text{current Na (mEq/L)/desired Na (mEq/L)}] - 1 \right)$$

For chronic hypernatremia, correction should be calculated to reduce the sodium by 10 mEq in a 24-hour period. The amount of water given in that period should also include any insensible and ongoing losses. Because too rapid a fall in sodium can result in brain swelling, follow-up laboratory monitoring of serum sodium every 4–6 hours is indicated. Patients who are volume overloaded may also benefit from the use of a thiazide diuretic.

Diabetes Insipidus

(Am Fam Physician 1997;55:2146)

Cause:

- Central diabetes insipidus: congenital; hypothalamic injury following brain trauma; Sheehan's syndrome
- Nephrogenic diabetes insipidus: hereditary; amphotericin B; demeclocycline; ethanol; foscarnet; lithium; hypercalcemia; kidney failure; ADPKD; postobstructive diuresis

Epidem: 10% of patients treated with long-term lithium therapy will develop irreversible nephrogenic diabetes insipidus (Drug Saf 1999;21:449).

Pathophys: ADH opens water channels (aquaporins) in the duct cells located in the distal tubule. In central diabetes insipidus, there is a defect in release of ADH from the hypothalamus. Hereditary nephrogenic diabetes insipidus is characterized by a mutation in the ADH receptor. Most cases of drug-induced nephrogenic diabetes insipidus and cases due to hypercalcemia are characterized by reduced number of aquaporins in the distal tubule. Amiloride can be a treatment for lithium-induced nephrogenic diabetes insipidus because it interferes with the uptake of lithium by the duct cells. This diminishes the polyuria due to lithium.

Sx: polyuria; polydipsia; nocturia

Crs: As long as water intake adequate, benign

Cmplc: hypernatremia

Labs: serum Na, serum osmolality, urine Na, urine osmolality, serum ADH level

If there is documented hypernatremia, administration of 0.4 mcg of ADH sc can distinguish central diabetes insipidus from nephrogenic diabetes insipidus. In central diabetes insipidus, the urine osmolality will rise by 100 mOsm/L or more after ADH is given.

For patients with polyuria and normal serum osmolality, a water deprivation test can distinguish primary polydipsia from central or nephrogenic diabetes insipidus.

Minimum 2-hour fast, measure initial serum Na, serum osmolality, urine osmolality, and serum ADH level.

Begin 4 hours of water deprivation; use hard candy to mitigate thirst; measure hourly: urine output, serum Na, serum osmolality, and urine osmolality.

The first phase of the test can be terminated if at any time (before or during test) the serum Na > 145 mEq/L, serum osmolality > 280 mOsm, or urine osmolality > 300 mOsm/L. A final ADH level is drawn at this time. If the urine osmolality < 300 after 4 hours, then 0.4 mcg of ADH is administered sc.

One hour after injection of ADH, measure final urine output, serum Na, serum osmolality, and urine osmolality (see Table 1.3).

Table 1.3   Interpretation of a Water Deprivation Test

Diagnosis	Serum Na	Urine Osm before ADH	Urine Osm after ADH	Urine Output	Initial ADH	Final ADH
Central diabetes insipidus	Rises to over 145 mEq/L	Always < 300 mOsm/L	Rises by more than 100 mOsm/L	Falls after ADH	Low	Low
Nephrogenic diabetes insipidus	Rises to over 145 mEq/L	Always < 300 mOsm/L	No change or rises < 100 mOsm/L	Always high	Variable	High
Primary polydipsia	Dose not go over 140 mEq/L	Rises during test to at least 300 mOsm/L		Decreases during water deprivation	Variable	High

1.3   Hypokalemia

Cause:

- Decreased intake: Obligate losses are only about 40 mEq/d, so this is almost always seen in conjunction with very poor overall nutritional intake.
- Extracellular to intracellular shifts: metabolic alkalosis, insulin, beta-agonists, hypokalemic periodic paralysis
- Increased losses: diuretics, distal renal tubular acidosis, Bartter's disorder, Gitelman's syndrome, mineralocorticoid excess (hyperaldosteronism), hypomagnesemia, diarrhea, vomiting
- Pseudohypokalemia: potassium movement into cells after blood drawn into tube

Epidem: Patients with eating disorders (Arch Intern Med 2005;165:561), alcoholics (Drug Alcohol Rev 2002;21:73), and patients taking thiazide diuretics or loop diuretics (Br Med J 1980;280:905) are groups at risk for hypokalemia.

Pathophys: Potassium is the major intracellular cation with a concentration of 140 mEq/L. This compares to the extracellular concentration of approximately 4 mEq/L. In a 70 kg individual, only 60 mEq of potassium is extracellular compared to approximately 4000 mEq of total potassium in the body. The extracellular potassium concentration is regulated not only by passage of potassium in and out of the individual but also by shifting potassium between intracellular and extracellular spaces. Several mechanisms are responsible for shifting potassium. Insulin and beta-adrenergic stimulation facilitate potassium movement into cells. Glucagon and alpha-adrenergic stimulation block this movement. The potassium gradient is also used to defend the intracellular acid-base status. In alkalosis, potassium ions are shifted intracellularly in exchange for hydrogen ions.

Urinary potassium loss is enhanced by aldosterone, which enhances the activity of a Na/K active transport ion exchanger located in the distal tubule. The ion exchanger is also activated by the delivery of sodium and water to the distal tubule. This accounts for the increased potassium loss caused by thiazide diuretics, loop diuretics, and osmotic agents. Urinary potassium excretion is also enhanced by alkalosis, where potassium is secreted into the urine in exchange for hydrogen ions. The channels that allow potassium to enter cells with the concentration gradient require magnesium for optimal function (J Physiol 1981;315:421). Magnesium deficiency decreases the passive reabsorption of potassium in the tubule.

Gastrointestinal losses from the colon and small intestine are on the order of 50–70 mEq/L; thus, large losses are often accompanied by hypokalemia. Upper gastrointestinal losses lead to hypokalemia through a number of these processes. The actual losses in the secretions are a modest 10 mEq/L, but urinary losses are significant. The volume depletion state stimulates the production of aldosterone, and the loss of hydrogen ion leads to alkalosis. Both processes enhance urinary potassium elimination.

Signs and symptoms of hypokalemia are due to changes in the resting membrane potential across the cell membrane. The large potassium gradient is an important determinant of the resting membrane potential. Hypokalemia increases the gradient which results in an increase in the resting membrane potential. This leads to disruption of the cardiac conduction system and muscle cell contraction.

Sx: Muscle weakness, cramps, palpitations, muscle pain

Si: Muscle weakness, diminished deep tendon reflexes, cardiac arrhythmias, rhabdomyolysis

Lab: Urine K, urine Na, urine Cl, urine osmolality, serum osmolality, electrolytes, BUN, creatinine, Mg, glu, EKG, CPK

The trans-tubular potassium gradient (TTKG) is an indicator of the kidneys' avidity to reabsorb potassium.

TTKG = (Urine K/Serum K)/(U osmolality/S osmolality)

The normal value is around 8 (see Table 1.4).

When the urine K is elevated (> 40 mEq/L, TTKG > 11) along with a high or normal serum bicarbonate, it is likely that aldosterone production is high. In the setting of hypovolemia, it is important to measure the other urinary electrolytes Na and Cl. The aldosterone production could be stimulated by gastrointestinal losses (urine Na < 20 mEq/L or urine Cl mEq/L < 20) or by overuse of diuretics (urine Na > 20 mEq/L and urine Cl > 20 mEq/L). With copious upper gastrointestinal losses, there is loss of bicarbonate in the urine. When that anion is lost, a cation must also be excreted. Often it is sodium, so under these circumstances a low urine Cl is a more sensitive marker of volume depletion than urine Na. An elevated urine K or TTKG accompanied by hypertension requires a different workup. Plasma renin

Table 1.4 Interpretation of Clinical Data in Hypokalemia

	TTKG	Urine K	Serum HCO3	Urine Na	Urine Cl	Hyper-tension
Inadequate intake	< 3	< 20 mEq/L	Normal			
Lower gastrointestinal losses	< 3	< 20 mEq/L	Low	< 20 mEq/L	< 20 mEq/L	No
Diuretic use without hypovolemia or hypomagnesemia	> 11	> 40 mEq/L	Normal	> 20 mEq/L	> 20 mEq/L	
Overuse of diuretics	> 11	> 40 mEq/L	High	> 20 mEq/L	> 20 mEq/L	No
Upper gastrointestinal losses	> 11	> 40 mEq/L	High		< 20 mEq/L	No
High aldosterone state with hypertension	> 11	> 40 mEq/L	Normal or high			Yes

activity, aldosterone levels, cortisol levels, and urinary steroid breakdown products are often measured. Renovascular hypertension is characterized by an elevated renin and aldosterone level (see Chapter 10.10). Adrenal hyperplasia is noted by the suppressed renin level and an elevated aldosterone level. Cushing's disease is noted by the high cortisol level, and defects in the corticosteroid synthesis are diagnosed by the elevated levels of urinary steroid breakdown products.

Rx: Several factors complicate the normalization of serum potassium levels. Because the majority of potassium is located in the intracellular compartment, it is hard to estimate the total body deficit based on the serum potassium level. The relatively small amount of potassium in the serum also means that iv administration can cause a rapid rise in serum potassium, which can lead to cardiac arrhythmias. In addition, potassium chloride is quite irritating to peripheral veins, which limits the concentrations that can be used. The safest way to replenish potassium is via the oral route. A potassium rich diet or oral potassium supplements can be used, and the potassium levels should be rechecked at least daily. In cases of hypokalemia associated with cardiac arrhythmia or where the risk of arrhythmia is high, iv administration of potassium chloride can be given while cardiac monitoring. IV supplementation at a rate of 10 mEq/hr can be given in a central vein as a solution of 40 mEq in 100 ml of normal saline. It can be given in peripheral vein at the same rate in a concentration of 40 mEq in 1000 ml of diluent. In this situation, the serum potassium should be measured after each 40 mEq. Oral repletion can be given at the same time. It is also important to mitigate any ongoing losses. This includes slowing any gastrointestinal losses, stopping loop and thiazide diuretics, and replacing magnesium if required. Strategies to prevent diuretic-induced hypokalemia include a diet rich in high potassium foods (Chest 2004;125:404) or adding potassium-sparing diuretics to the regimen.

Bartter's Syndrome

Cause: A rare autosomal recessive cause of hypokalemia. The genetic defect is in the Na-K-2Cl ion cotransporter in the thick ascending limb of the loop of Henle (J Am Soc Nephrol 2003;14:1419).

Pathophys: The phenotype is characterized by hypokalemia, metabolic alkalosis, hypercalciuria, and activation of aldosterone without hypertension. The phenotypical kidney physiology mimics the effect of loop diuretics on the kidney. Several genotypes have been identified. Some cause defects in the synthesis of the transporter, and another is in a helper protein that inserts the transporter into the plasma membrane (Nephron 2002;92[suppl 1]:18).

Sx: Polyuria, polydipsia, muscle cramps

Crs: Some genotypes are associated with mental retardation and growth failure; others are associated with deafness. Usually diagnosed in the neonatal period or early childhood.

Lab: Electrolytes, Mg, serum aldosterone level, urine K, urine Na, urine Cl, 24-hour urine for K and Ca

Hypokalemia, hypochloremia, and an elevated serum bicarbonate are the typical serum findings. Hypomagnesemia and elevated aldosterone levels are also present. Urinary findings include elevated levels of K, Cl, and Ca. The syndrome can be differentiated from surreptitious vomiting by the elevated urine Cl. Other than the fact that this is almost never diagnosed in adulthood, the only way to exclude surreptitious diuretic or laxative use is to perform urinary screens for these medications.

Rx: Potassium supplements, potassium rich diet, and NSAIDs

Gitelman's Syndrome

Cause: A rare autosomal recessive cause of hypokalemia. Sometimes it is characterized as a variant of Bartter's syndrome, but the defective ion transporter is located in the distal tubule (N Engl J Med 1999;340:1177).

Pathophys: Like Bartter's syndrome, hypokalemia, metabolic alkalosis, and activation of aldosterone are present; however, since the defective transporter is located in the distal tubule, hypocalciuria is present rather than hypercalciuria. The kidney physiology of Gitelman's syndrome mimics the effect of thiazide diuretics on the kidney.

Sx: Polyuria, polydipsia, muscle cramps

Lab: Electrolytes, Mg, serum aldosterone level, urine K, urine Na, urine Cl, 24-hour urine for K and Ca

Hypokalemia, hypochloremia, and an elevated serum bicarbonate are the typical serum findings. Hypomagnesemia and elevated aldosterone levels are also present. Urinary findings include elevated levels of K and Cl but below normal Ca. The syndrome can be differentiated from surreptitious vomiting by the elevated urine Cl. Often, the only way to differentiate Gitelman's syndrome from surreptitious thiazide diuretic use or laxative use is to perform urinary screens for these medications.

Rx: Potassium supplements, potassium-rich diet, and NSAIDs

1.4   Hyperkalemia

Cause:

- Increased intake: There are many dietary sources rich in potassium, including citrus fruits, dried fruits, nuts, dairy, protein rich meat, and dark colored vegetables. Potassium-containing salt substitutes contain approximately 7 mEq in a 1 g serving. Normal potassium homeostasis allows for considerable dietary intake, so cases of hyperkalemia from increased intake are almost always accompanied by a defect in potassium excretion.

- Intracellular to extracellular shifts: In rhabdomyolysis, tumor lysis syndrome, intravascular hemolysis, or other tissue breakdown, the potassium is released directly from compromised cells. Acidosis, hyperosmolar states, and succinylcholine stimulate the movement of potassium out of the cell. Digoxin, insulin deficiency, and beta-agonist blockade all hinder the entry of potassium into the cell.
- Decreased excretion: Kidney failure, distal renal tubular acidosis, hypoaldosteronism
- Pseudohyperkalemia: This occurs when potassium is released from cells after the blood has been drawn. Fist-clenching during blood draw, thrombocytosis, and severe leukocytosis can be responsible.

Epidem:

Risk factors:

- ACEI use
- CKD
- Cardiac disease (Am Heart J 2006;152:705): CHF Class III or IV, Afib
- Diabetes mellitus: As many as 15% of diabetics presenting for a diabetic clinic visit have K > 5 mEq/L (BMJ 2003;327:812).

   Recent trends in medication therapy impact in the incidence of hyperkalemia. As an example, hyperkalemia admission rates went from 2.3/1000 hospitalized patients in 1994 to 11/1000 hospitalized patients in 2001 following the RALES study, where spironolactone was added to ACEI for the treatment of CHF (N Engl J Med 2004;351:543).

Pathophys: See Chapter 1.3 for a discussion of potassium homeostasis; also see Table 1.5.

Table 1.5 Mechanisms for Drug-Induced Hyperkalemia

Drug	Mechanism
Potassium supplements	Increased intake
Spironolactone, eplerenone	Blocks aldosterone
Amiloride	Blocks Na-K transporter in the distal renal tubule principal cells
Triamterene	Blocks Na-K transporter in the distal renal tubule principal cells
Heparin	Interferes with aldosterone synthesis
Beta blockers	Slow potassium shift into cells and block renin and aldosterone release
ACEIs	Block renin and aldosterone release and decrease GFR
ARBs	Block renin and aldosterone release and decrease GFR
NSAIDs	Decrease GFR, renin, and aldosterone levels
Digoxin	Blocks Na/K ATPase (decrease potassium shift into cells)
Succinylcholine	Depolarize cell membrane; potassium moves out of cells
TMP-SX	Blocks Na-K transporter in the distal renal tubule principal cells

Several factors make diabetics especially prone to hyperkalemia. Diabetic dietary advice often relies on food groups high in potassium. Excretion may be limited by kidney failure, ACEI, or ARB use and hypoaldosteronism. Potassium entry into cells is diminished by insulin deficiency. Shifts of potassium out of cells are seen in hyperosmolar states associated with hyperglycemia and with diabetic ketoacidosis.

Sx: Muscle weakness

Si: Cardiac arrhythmias

Lab: Rule out pseudohyperkalemia; hemolysis is likely if a plasma potassium measured in a heparinized blood sample is more than 0.5 mEq/L lower than the serum value.

The trans-tubular potassium gradient (TTKG) is an indicator of the kidney's avidity to reabsorb potassium. The normal value is around 8.

$$TTKG = (Urine\ K/Serum\ K)/$$
$$(Urine\ osmolality/Serum\ osmolality).$$

When hyperkalemia is present, if the TTKG < 5, a defect in renal potassium excretion is present. Hypoaldosteronism or kidney failure is usually responsible.

Xray: EKG changes (in order of increasing alarm):
- Peaked T-waves
- Prolonged QRS
- Loss of P-wave
- Sine wave
- Ventricular fibrillation

Rx: When hyperkalemia is associated with muscle weakness, EKG changes, or the serum K > 7 mEq/L, stabilization of the cell membrane is indicated. 10–20 mEq of calcium chloride (10–20 ml of 10% calcium chloride solution or 10% calcium gluconate solution) is given intravenously over 5–10 min. The effect of calcium on the cell membrane is temporary, and administration can be repeated. Calcium should not be given to patients on digoxin. The next step is to lower the serum potassium by taking advantage of cellular shifts. Glucose 50 g iv followed by 10 units of regular insulin will enhance potassium movement into cells. Nebulizer treatment with albuterol or levalbuterol will acutely lower the serum K (Emerg Med J 2005;22:366). Intravenous sodium bicarbonate is reserved for cases where the hyperkalemia is accompanied by acidosis. Once these steps have been accomplished and for less severe hyperkalemia (5.5 mEq/L < K < 7 mEq/L), the next goal is elimination of potassium. Loop and thiazide diuretic enhance renal excretion. Hemodialysis is very effective for removing potassium directly from the plasma. Sodium polystyrene sulfonate is a cation exchange resin that will exchange Na for K in the gastrointestinal tract. The usual dose is 15–60 g either orally or rectally. Although a single dose is no more effective than cathartics for the treatment of acute hyperkalemia (J Am Soc Nephrol 1998;9:1924), doses of 5–15 g daily are effective for the treatment of chronic hyperkalemia. Prevention of hyperkalemia is important to consider in the high risk groups, including those with diabetes, chronic kidney disease, and congestive heart failure. Dietary consultation for a low potassium diet, avoidance of spironolactone and other potassium-sparing diuretics for patients with creatinine > 2 mg/dL or GFR < 30 ml/min/1.73 m^2, and avoidance of NSAIDs for patients on ACEI or ARB are effective strategies (N Engl J Med 2004;351:585).

1.5 Hypocalcemia

(Best Pract Res Clin Endocrinol Metab 2003;17:623)

Cause:

- Kidney failure
- Hypoparathyroidism
- Pseudohypoparathyroidism
- Post-thyroidectomy
- Malabsorption
- Vitamin D deficiency
- Rhabdomyolysis
- Pancreatitis
- Bisphosphonates
- Massive blood transfusion
- Gadolinium administration for MRI

- Hypomagnesemia
- Cinacalcet
- Anticonvulsant therapy

Epidem: 25%–35% of patients undergoing total thyroidectomy will experience transient hypocalcemia (Otolaryngol Head Neck Surg 2007;136:278).

Pathophys: Several mechanisms are responsible for hypocalcemia.

- Parathyroid hormone deficiency can be due to surgical removal or immunologic failure of the glands.
- Cinacalcet decreases the sensitivity of the parathyroid gland to low calcium levels.
- Magnesium is required for PTH secretion.
- Pseudohypoparathyroidism is due to end organ resistance to PTH.
- Vitamin D deficiency can be due to inadequate intake, inadequate exposure to sunlight, or kidney failure. The kidney adds a 1-hydroxl group to 25(OH) vitamin D, which creates the most biologically active form of the vitamin.
- Several anticonvulsants, including phenytoin, carbamazepine, and phenobarbital, stimulate microsomal enzymes that enhance the breakdown of vitamin D (Neurology 2002;58:1348).
- Chelation of calcium with dietary fats can occur in the gastrointestinal tract in patients with malabsorption syndromes. Chelation of calcium occurs in the bloodstream from the release of fatty acids in severe pancreatitis, by EDTA used to preserve blood, and by gadolinium administered for MRI.
- In rhabdomyolysis, calcium binds to the phosphorous released by the damaged muscle tissue.
- Several medications will block the release of calcium from bone, including bisphosphonates, calcitonin, and gallium nitrate.

The symptoms of hypocalcemia are due to neuromuscular irritability. The low extracellular concentration decreases the threshold for depolarization by enhancing membrane permeability to sodium.

Sx: Perioral and distal extremity numbness or tingling; muscle cramps

Si:

- Carpal pedal spasms
- Tetany
- Seizures
- Trousseau sign: Inflate brachial blood pressure cuff above the systolic BP for several minutes. The ischemia will enhance the nerves excitability, and carpal spasms can be elicited.
- Chvostek sign: The enhanced excitability of the facial nerve can be demonstrated by physical stimulation of the nerve as it exits the external auditory meatus. 10% of normal individuals may have a positive Chvostek's sign.

Lab: Serum albumin, ionized calcium, Mg, PTH, 25 (OH) vitamin D, 1,25 (OH) vitamin D

Rule out factitious hypocalcemia in patients with hypoalbuminemia. The physiologically important calcium concentration is the ionized calcium. The standard measured calcium level is the total calcium concentration. Each gram of albumin in the blood binds approximately 0.8 mg of calcium. Where serum albumin is measured in g/dL, and calcium is measured in mg/dL, the following equation will correct for low serum albumin levels:

$$\text{Corrected calcium} = \text{measured calcium} + (0.8 \times (4 - \text{serum albumin})),$$

Acidosis will decrease the number of binding sites on proteins for calcium, and alkalosis increases the number of binding sites. Because of the many variables that can determine the ionized calcium, it can be very helpful to measure the ionized calcium directly, especially in the critically ill patient (Crit Care Med 2003;31:1389). PTH levels and levels of 25 (OH) vitamin D and 1,25 (OH) vitamin D should be measured when the diagnosis is in doubt. Magnesium should be measured, as treatment will be less effective if hypomagnesemia is not corrected.

Rx: Mild hypocalcemia can be treated with oral calcium supplementation. Calcium carbonate and calcium citrate have been shown to be equally effective. Vitamin D supplementation is also advised. For patients with chronic kidney disease, 1,25 (OH) vitamin D (calcitriol) or a vitamin D analog should be administered. For symptomatic hypocalcemia, iv calcium can be administered. 10% calcium gluconate (10 ml ampules) or 10% calcium chloride (10 ml) can be given acutely. The calcium chloride ampules contain more elemental calcium per ml, but the solution can be irritating to the vein. An iv solution of 100 ml of 10% calcium gluconate in 1 L of normal saline or D5W can be administered over 10–12 hours with serial monitoring of calcium concentration every 4 hours.

1.6   Hypercalcemia

(Crit Care Med 2004;32:S146)

Cause:

- Hyperparathyroidism
- Malignancy
- Thiazide diuretics
- Vitamin D intoxication
- Milk-alkali syndrome
- Immobilization
- Granulomatous diseases including sarcoidosis, tuberculosis, and pulmonary fungal infections

Epidem: Population studies show that malignancy and primary hyper-parathyroidism are the 2 most common causes of hypercalcemia. 7.5% of patients presenting to an emergency room had hyper-calcemia; malignancy was the highest single cause, accounting for 36% of the cases of elevated calcium. It was noted that over 75% of the patients that presented with hypercalcemia also had impaired kidney function (Am J Med Sci 2006;331:119).

Pathophys: The serum calcium is regulated by the parathyroid hormone interacting with the target organs of the kidneys and the bones. Additional feedback in the system is provided by Vitamin D and its target organs: the gastrointestinal tract and the parathyroid glands. A drop in serum calcium stimulates PTH release. This increases bone resorption and decreases renal calcium excretion. It also stimulates the kidney to produce active vitamin D. 1,25 (OH) vitamin D provides negative feedback on the parathyroid gland and increases calcium absorption from the gastrointestinal tract.

Hypercalcemia has several effects on the kidney. Acute manifestations include nephrogenic diabetes insipidus caused by a decrease in the number of aquaporins in the distal tubule. Acute kidney injury is due to renal vasoconstriction. Systemic vasoconstriction and the positive inotropic effect of hypercal-cemia contribute to hypertension. A common clinical scenario is hypercalcemia accompanied by acute kidney injury, volume depletion, hypernatremia, and hypertension. Chronic hypercal-cemia is a risk factor for nephrolithiasis.

Sx: Lethargy; weakness; polyuria, polydipsia, constipation

Si: Weakness, confusion, hyporeflexia

Labs: PTH; 25 (OH) vitamin D; 1,25 (OH) vitamin D; alkaline phos-phatase; TSH; search for underlying malignancy, which could include the PSA level, SPEP

Xray: Search for underlying malignancy, which could include the following:

- CXR
- Bone survey
- Bone scan
- Mammograms

Rx: Mild cases (Ca < 11.5 mg/dL) are treated by looking for the underlying cause and eliminating or treating it. More serious cases require attempts to reduce the serum calcium. It is important to initially assess the patient's volume status and kidney function. If the patient can establish urine flow, then excretion of excess calcium by the kidneys can be attempted. First of all, any volume deficit should be corrected with normal saline. Once the patient is euvolemic, iv furosemide or other loop diuretics should be used to establish a calcium diuresis. In cases where kidney failure is not easily reversed, dialysis is also effective at lowering serum calcium.

The serum calcium can also be reduced by blocking bone resorption with bisphosphonates, gallium nitrate, or calcitonin. Calcitonin is given 4 unit/kg sc or im every 12 hours. It should be noted that the effect of calcitonin is short lived, thus only a few days of therapy are indicated. On the other hand, bisphosphonates are quite effective for long-term suppression of calcium, but they have a slower onset of action. IV pamidronate, zoledronic acid, and ibandronate are all effective for lowering serum calcium. Nephrotoxicity is a concern with long-term use of bisphosphonates, including the nephritic syndrome with pamidronate and acute kidney injury with zoledronic acid. Gallium nitrate is an option for resistant cases, although nephrotoxicity is also its major adverse reaction (Semin Oncol 2003;30:13).

1.7   Hypomagnesemia

Causes:

- Inadequate intake
- Increased urinary losses: diuretics, renal tubular damage or disorders (aminoglycosides, cisplatin, amphotericin B, cyclosporine, postobstructive diuresis)
- Increased gastrointestinal losses: nasogastric drainage; laxatives
- Increased tissue uptake: refeeding after starvation

Epidem: Several population studies point to a surprisingly high prevalence of this disorder including 14.7% in unselected populations (Magnes Res 2001;14:283). 31% in patients presenting to the ER (Am J Emerg Med 2003;21:444), and 20% in an urban clinic with a population predominantly African American and female (J Fam Pract 1999;48:636).

Pathophys: High delivery of sodium to the distal tubule or distal tubular damage will inhibit the reabsorption of magnesium performed in the distal tubule. Because magnesium is an important cofactor in the function of Na/K exchangers in the distal tubule, hypokalemia is a complication of magnesium deficiency. It is also a cofactor for the release of PTH from the parathyroid glands and is associated with hypocalcemia. Magnesium deficiency is also implicated in a number of disease processes, including hypertension and the metabolic syndrome (J Hypertens 2000;18:1177).

Sx: Weakness, seizures

Si: Ventricular arrhythmias

Cmplc: Hypokalemia, hypocalcemia

Lab: If the reason for magnesium deficiency is in doubt, a 24-hour urine for magnesium can be collected. In magnesium deficiency, the kidneys should excrete no more than 12 mg (0.5 mmol) in 24 hours.

Rx: Oral replacement; dietary sources include green vegetables, nuts, and seeds. Several magnesium salts, including magnesium oxide and magnesium gluconate, are also available, but the side effect of oral administration of these is diarrhea; thus, dosing is limited.

Intravenous magnesium sulfate is an option for hospitalized patients. The dosing is 1 g iv every 12 hours. It is important to write "magnesium sulfate" rather than to use the chemical formula abbreviation ($MgSO4$) in order to avoid confusion with morphine sulfate.

1.8 Total Body Sodium Excess and Diuretic Therapy of Edema

(N Engl J Med 1998;339:387)

Introduction: Retention of dietary sodium and water and subsequent capillary leak of fluid into tissues causes edema. Common edematous states lead to a generalized increase in total body sodium and water. Differing properties of various capillary and lymphatic beds may lead some patients to present with local findings such as lower extremity edema or pulmonary edema. Less commonly, edema due to localized lymphatic or venous obstruction in a single limb will be present. In these unusual cases, most of the patient's body has a normal sodium and water content, and the edematous limb requires local treatment only.

Diuretics are commonly used in clinical practice for the treatment of the following edematous conditions:

- Left heart failure and cardiogenic pulmonary edema
- Fluid retention due to acute or chronic kidney disease
- Cirrhosis with ascites
- Nephrotic syndrome

The following general principles apply to diuretic therapy of these conditions:

- Loop diuretics are most commonly utilized for the treatment of edema. These drugs are excreted into the tubular lumen where they reach their site of action. Kidney impairment leads to prolongation of the furosemide but not the bumetanide or torsemide half-life.
- Dietary sodium restriction is a critical aspect of successful diuretic therapy. Diuretic-resistant patients who are not on sodium-restricted diets may be unable to achieve adequate diuresis due to high sodium intake.
- Any time diuretics are prescribed care should be taken to avoid undue volume depletion and circulatory collapse.
- Ethacrinic acid is available for patients who are allergic to furosemide and bumetanide. Ethacrinic acid is more ototoxic than the other loop diuretics, and its use should be limited to patients who are unable to take other loop diuretics.
- Loop diuretics only elicit a response once the critical threshold concentration is reached at the site of action. Failure to respond to a dose of a loop diuretic should be followed by dose escalation until an effective (above the threshold) dose is found. The maximum iv one-time dose of furosemide and bumetanide is 240 mg and 6 mg, respectively, every 6 hours. Maximum oral doses of loop diuretics are usually about twice the iv dose. Some patients have unpredictable absorption of loop diuretics that may be due to bowel edema.
- Patients who respond to bolus doses of loop diuretics but are unable to achieve adequate net diuresis can be treated with continuous infusions. Continuous infusions should only be used in patients who have an adequate response to bolus doses. The aim of the infusion is to continuously maintain the concentration of the loop diuretic above the threshold level at the site of action. The same total daily dose of a diuretic administered as a bolus followed by continuous infusion will produce a greater net diuresis than if that dose were administered

intermittently. This phenomenon is due to the drop of the diuretic concentration below the threshold level at the site of action at the end of the dosing interval.

- Chronic administration of loop diuretics leads to hypertrophy of the thiazide sensitive portion of the nephron. This allows sodium reabsorption in that segment that diminishes loop diuretic effectiveness. Administration of thiazide diuretics, such as daily oral metolazone or intravenous chlorothiazide, can reduce loop diuretic resistance in many patients.

- In patients with nephrotic syndrome and severe hypoalbuminemia, diuretics may not reach the site of action due to being bound to the pathologically filtered albumin in the tubular lumen. For this reason, higher diuretic doses are usually required.

- Patients with cirrhosis should be placed on adequate doses of spironolactone, which should be titrated to at least 200 mg daily. If adequate diuresis cannot be achieved with spironolactone alone, a loop diuretic can be added.

- Patients with CHF are usually treated with loop diuretics. In these patients, more frequent administration of loop diuretics leads to greater net diuresis. Spironolactone has been shown to improve survival of patients with severe heart failure (N Engl J Med 1999;341:709).

- Spironolactone should not be administered to patients with GFR below 30 ml/min due to increased risk of severe hyperkalemia.

- Patients with metabolic alkalosis, including contraction alkalosis, can be treated with acetazolamide, which produces urinary bicarbonate loss.

- Patients with cor pulmonale can be treated with loop diuretics, but the treatment may be limited by volume depletion and hypotension. Treatment of the underlying lung disorder should include treatment of hypercapnia and hypoxia. In some patients, pulmonary vasodilators may be appropriate. Acetazolamide may be particularly useful in these patients who may respond to an increase in arterial pH with worsening hypoventilation.

Chapter 2

Acid-Base Disorders

2.1 Approach to a Patient with an Acid-Base Disorder

(Postgrad Med 2000;107:249)
Often the first indication of an acid-base disorder is a finding of abnormal serum bicarbonate during laboratory testing.

- Start with a history and physical. The underlying illness will often offer a clue to the diagnosis of an underlying acid-base disturbance.
- Obtain an ABG simultaneously with serum electrolytes.
- Do not rely on the serum bicarbonate to make a diagnosis in an incompletely understood case. Remember that elevated serum bicarbonate can be seen in both metabolic alkalosis and chronic respiratory acidosis. Similarly, low serum bicarbonate can be seen in metabolic acidosis and chronic respiratory alkalosis.
- Calculate the anion gap.

$$\text{Anion gap} = (Na) - ([Cl] + [HCO_3])$$

- A patient with an elevated anion gap always has a metabolic acidosis, and the cause is usually ascertainable when the anion gap is above 20 even when the serum bicarbonate is normal or high.

- The differential diagnosis of elevated anion gap metabolic acidosis includes a number of poisonings and intoxications where a rapid diagnosis and initiation of treatment is required for a good outcome. These include salicylate, ethylene glycol, and methanol poisoning, along with others. Laboratory tests for the salicylate level are widely available. Determination of ethylene glycol and methanol levels can require a prolonged time period. Calculation of the osmolar gap allows for rapid ascertainment of the presence of exogenous osmoles in these cases. A calculated osmolar gap of greater than 10 mOsm/L (measured osmolality exceeds calculated osmolality by more than 10) may suggest a poisoning with an agent such as ethylene glycol, methanol, or other alcohols or solvents.

$$\text{Osmolar gap} = \text{serum osmolality} - (2x\ Na^+ + glucose/180 + BUN/2.8 + ethanol/4.6)$$

- In cases of respiratory acidosis, for each 10 mm Hg increase in pCO_2, expect a 1 mEq/L increase in serum bicarbonate in acute respiratory acidosis and 3 mEq/L in chronic respiratory acidosis.
- Once the arterial blood gas and serum electrolyte results are available, determine the primary disorder. Compensatory mechanisms do not correct the pH all the way back to normal; therefore, the disturbance most consistent with the deviation in pH will usually be the primary disorder (eg, low pH and low bicarbonate are consistent with primary metabolic acidosis, while low pH and high pCO_2 will usually signify that respiratory acidosis is the primary disorder).
- If the anion gap or serum bicarbonate is significantly abnormal and the pH is normal, then 2 primary disorders are likely present.

- If metabolic acidosis is present, use Winter's formula to calculate the pCO_2 expected for a patient with a given serum bicarbonate and normal respiratory compensation (Ann Intern Med 1967;66:312).

$$\text{Expected } pCO_2 = HCO_3 \times 1.5 + 8$$

- If the expected pCO_2 is within 2 mm Hg of the measured pCO_2, the appropriate respiratory compensation to the metabolic disorder is present. If the expected pCO_2 is higher than the measured pCO_2, then the respiratory compensation is inadequate and concurrent respiratory acidosis is present. This finding may herald impending respiratory failure due to respiratory muscle fatigue. If the expected pCO_2 is lower than measured, then a concurrent respiratory alkalosis is present.
- In respiratory acidosis, for each 10 mm Hg increase in pCO_2, expect a 1 mEq/L increase in serum bicarbonate in acute respiratory acidosis and 3 mEq/L in chronic respiratory acidosis.
- In respiratory alkalosis, for each 10 mm Hg increase in pCO_2, expect a 2 mEq/L decrease in serum bicarbonate in acute respiratory alkalosis and 5 mEq/L in chronic respiratory alkalosis.

2.2 Metabolic Acidosis

(Rose, Post; Clinical Physiology of Acid-Base and Electrolyte Disorders, New York; McGraw-Hill, 2001; Emerg Med Clin North Am 2005;23:771)

Introduction: Three mechanisms can lead to metabolic acidosis: increased acid production, loss of bicarbonate in urine or via the gastrointestinal tract, and impaired renal excretion of acid in renal failure. The diagnosis of metabolic acidosis requires the measurement of both arterial blood pH and serum bicarbonate concentration. Decreased serum bicarbonate alone can be seen in metabolic acidosis and in chronic respiratory alkalosis. Measurement of pCO_2 is required to assess the degree of respiratory compensation. Calculation of the anion gap is useful for the differential diagnosis of metabolic acidosis.

$$Anion\ gap = (Na) - ([Cl] + [HCO_3])$$

The normal anion gap is 5–11 mEq/L and is dependent on the normal ranges for electrolytes, which can differ among labs (Arch Intern Med 1990;150:311). Hypocalcemia, hypokalemia, and hypomagnesemia will produce a decreased anion gap. Hypoalbuminemia requires a downward adjustment of the normal anion gap by 2.5 mEq/L for every 1 g/dL reduction in serum albumin concentration (Kidney Int 1985;27:472). In patients with severe hypoalbuminemia, multiplying serum albumin by 3 produces a reasonable approximation of the expected anion gap. Newer data suggest that the "normal" anion gap value is lower than 12 mEq/L when electrolytes are measured using modern laboratory equipment (Arch Intern Med 1990;150:311).When the anion gap is above 25 mEq/L, the diagnosis of one of the conditions described below is very likely to be made. It is not always possible to identify the unmeasured anion when the anion gap is elevated to a lesser degree (N Engl J Med 1980;303:854).

2.3   Elevated Anion Gap Metabolic Acidosis

Introduction: Calculation of the anion gap should be undertaken whenever an acidosis is recognized. Elevated anion gap metabolic acidosis includes a number of emergent medical conditions, which require prompt recognition and treatment. The mnemonic device MUDPILES is traditionally used as a memory aid for the differential diagnosis of elevated anion gap metabolic acidosis.

Methanol poisoning

Uremia

Diabetic ketoacidosis and starvation and alcoholic ketoacidosis

Pyroglutamic acidosis and Paraldehyde poisoning

Iron poisoning, Isoniazid poisoning

Lactic acidosis

Ethylene glycol poisoning

Salicylate poisoning

Several of the more important causes of elevated anion gap metabolic acidosis are described next.

Lactic Acidosis

Cause: The most common causes of lactic acidosis are tissue hypoperfusion and ischemia. Inadequate oxygen delivery can be seen in cases of inadequate tissue oxygen delivery due to severe anemia or carbon monoxide poisoning. Type A lactic acidosis is caused by shock, while type B lactic acidosis is due to regional ischemia. D-lactic acidosis occurs due to generation of D-lactate by colon bacteria. Lactic acidosis has been described in the absence of hypoxia in patients with HIV (Ann Intern Med 1993;118:37). Metformin therapy in patients with renal failure is a rare but frequently emphasized cause of lactic acidosis.

Pathophys:

- Type A lactic acidosis is usually caused by generalized tissue hypoperfusion due to:
  - Any form of shock or cardiac arrest
  - Severe hypoxemia
  - Severe anemia
  - Carbon monoxide poisoning
- Type B lactic acidosis occurs when generalized tissue perfusion is adequate, but there is either regional hypoperfusion or toxin-induced impairment of metabolism or mitochondrial function due to:

- Cyanide poisoning
- Metformin or phenformin (Diabetes Care 1999;22:925, Crit Care Med 2000;28:1803)
- Salicylate poisoning
- Propofol infusion (Anesthesiology 2004;101:239)
- Malignancy (Cancer 2001;92:2237, N Engl J Med 1980;303:1100)
- HIV infection
- HIV treatment with stavudine or didanosine (Ann Intern Med 1993;118:37) (Am J Nephrol 2000;20:332)
- D-lactate acidosis occurs after small bowel bypass or resection and is due to metabolism of carbohydrates by the bacteria in the colon to D-lactate, which, after absorption into the systemic circulation, is not recognized by L-lactate dehydrogenase (Kidney Int 1996;49:1)

Sx/Si: Usually related to the underlying disorder. Changes in pulmonary, cardiovascular, and neurologic function may occur. Shortness of breath, due to compensatory hyperventilation, and hyperpnea may be present.

Crs: Will depend on the cause of the underlying condition.

Cmplc: Very low arterial pH (< 7.1) can cause potentially fatal ventricular arrhythmias.

Lab: Serum lactate level, ABG, electrolytes, BUN, Cr, Mg, Ca, albumin, labs to rule out other causes of anion gap metabolic acidosis are usually necessary.

Rx: Treatment of the underlying condition that leads to inadequate tissue oxygenation such as hypoperfusion and shock with volume resuscitation and/or vasoactive therapy will lead to the improvement of the acidosis. Appropriate therapy for anemia and carbon monoxide poisoning will lead to resolution of the acidosis related to those conditions. In cases of metformin induced lactic acidosis, hemodialysis can be used to remove residual metformin. Hemodialysis alone is generally not effective for the treatment of lactic acidosis because in most cases the rate of clearance of lactate by dialysis is far below its rate of generation. Intractable lactic acidosis due to salicylate poisoning is described next.

Pyroglutamic Acidosis

(Clin Chem 1998;44:1497, Am J Kidney Dis 2005;46:143)

Cause: Pyroglutamic acid (5-oxoproline) accumulation (inherited due to glutathione synthase deficiency or acquired due to acetaminophen use) (Crit Care Med 2000;28:1803, Scand J Clin Lab Invest 1970;26:327).

Epidem: Acquired cases of pyroglutamic acidosis are usually seen in malnourished patients with sepsis who have previously ingested therapeutic or above therapeutic quantities of acetaminophen. Pyroglutamic acidosis can also be caused by a genetic deficiency of the enzymes glutathione synthase or 5-oxoprolinase. Not every patient with these genetic conditions will present with acidosis.

Pathophys: Treatment with acetaminophen leads to glutathione depletion. Under normal conditions, glutathione will be regenerated from cysteine. Under certain circumstances that often involve sepsis, malnutrition, prior acetaminophen ingestion, and renal failure, glutathione synthase activity is diminished and accumulation of 5-oxoproline will occur.

Sx/Si: Usually related to underlying sepsis, malnutrition and renal failure.

Crs: Related to the course of the underlying illness.

Lab: Consider testing for elevated urinary level of 5-oxoproline when the anion responsible for elevated anion gap cannot be identified.

Rx: Treat underlying sepsis and malnutrition; consider N-acetylcysteine therapy.

Diabetic Ketoacidosis

(Emerg Med Clin North Am 2005;23:609)

Cause: Absolute or relative insulinopenia due to lack of insulin therapy in Type 1 diabetes or inadequate supply of insulin in the setting of increased physiologic stress due to conditions such as sepsis, myocardial infarction, or any other severe illness. Ketoacidosis can also be seen in starvation and alcoholism.

Epidem: This condition usually occurs in individuals with Type 1 diabetes.

Pathophys: DKA occurs due to a relative deficiency of insulin and excess of insulin counter-regulatory hormones. Acidosis occurs once the body's ability to buffer ketone bodies (acetoacetate and β-hydroxybutyrate), which are weak acids, is overwhelmed by their production. Ketone bodies are produced by lipolysis of fatty acids.

Sx: Nausea and vomiting are often present. Other symptoms may be present due to the underlying illness that led to DKA.

Si: Exam will be consistent with volume depletion. Classic fruity smell of ketone bodies can be noted.

Crs: This condition is fatal if not promptly treated. Acidosis, volume depletion, and electrolyte depletion, particularly hypokalemia, can be very severe.

Cmplc: Hypovolemic shock, arrhythmias due to severe acidosis, and electrolyte disturbances.

Lab: Ketones will be present in urine and serum along with elevated anion gap metabolic acidosis. Initial hyperkalemia is common. This is followed by hypokalemia soon after volume repletion and insulin initiation. Magnesium and phosphorous depletion are also common. Unless non-compliance with insulin is clearly the cause of DKA, a work-up for conditions such as infection or myocardial infarction that may have caused DKA are indicated.

Rx: Volume repletion and administration of insulin by iv infusion are the initial therapies. Intravenous IV repletion of potassium, magnesium, and phosphate is often required. Underlying conditions such as infection or myocardial infarction may require simultaneous therapy. Sodium bicarbonate treatment should be reserved for patients with severe complications such as cardiac arrhythmias in the setting of very low pH.

Starvation and Alcoholic Ketoacidosis

Cause: Starvation, alcoholism in combination with starvation, nausea, and vomiting

Pathophys: Starvation can lead to insulin deficiency and glucagon and catecholamine excess leading to lipolysis of fatty acids and formation of ketone bodies. Because some insulin will be produced, the acidemia will not be as severe as that seen in DKA. Catecholamine surges seen with alcohol withdrawal will accelerate lipolysis and ketone body production and lead to more severe acidosis than that seen with starvation alone.

Lab: Ketones will be present in urine and serum along with elevated anion gap metabolic acidosis.

Rx: Supportive care with volume expansion with saline and dextrose and appropriate nutrition should be provided. Alcoholics should receive thiamine 100 mg iv or im to decrease the risk of Wernicke's or Korsakoff's syndrome.

Ethylene Glycol and Methanol Poisoning

(J Toxicol Clin Toxicol 2002;40:415)

Cause: Intentional or accidental ingestion of antifreeze or windshield washer fluid or other industrial products.

Epidem: In the developed world, deliberate suicide attempt is the most common cause of toxic ingestions. The majority of cases of accidental ingestion occur in children.

Pathophys: Once absorbed, these compounds are metabolized by hepatic alcohol dehydrogenase, which leads to accumulation of formate with methanol ingestion and accumulation of glycolate and oxalate with ethylene glycol ingestion. These metabolites are responsible for the clinical manifestations of these toxic ingestions.

Sx/Si: Patients with these overdoses will often present critically ill. Hyponatremia and seizures may occur. Methanol poisoning causes vision loss, which may or may not be present at the time of presentation. Shortness of breath, due to compensatory hyperventilation, and hyperpnea may be present.

Crs: Can be fatal if untreated.

Cmplc: Progression to end stage renal disease may occur in severe cases of ethylene glycol ingestion. Irreversible blindness is common with methanol ingestion.

Lab: Elevated anion gap metabolic acidosis can be present at presentation. Hyperosmolar hyponatremia may be present at presentation and finding of elevated osmolar gap may be present. Osmolar gap in excess of 10 mOsm/L is suggestive of the presence of a significant amount of an unmeasured osmotically active substance that may be a poison (J Toxicol Clin Toxicol 1993;31:81).

$$\text{Osmolar gap} = \text{serum osmolality} - (2\text{x [Na]} + \text{glucose}/180 + \text{BUN}/2.8 + \text{ethanol}/4.6)$$

Simultaneous presence of hyperosmolality or hyperosmolar hyponatremia and elevated anion gap metabolic acidosis should raise the suspicion of methanol or ethylene glycol poisoning. Measurement of blood levels of methanol and ethylene glycol may not be available emergently at all laboratories.

Rx: All poisoned patients require rapid assessment and stabilization of the airway, breathing, and circulation, along with identification of the poison followed by specific management. Ingestions of methanol or ethylene glycol should be treated with fomepizole or ethanol if fomepizole is not available, as well as emergent hemodialysis. These patients should also receive folic acid, thiamine, and pyridoxine. Patients with severe acidemia (arterial pH < 7.0) may be treated with sodium bicarbonate in order to prevent ventricular arrhythmias. The decision to treat must be made quickly based on history, high index of suspicion, and limited laboratory data.

Salicylate Poisoning

Cause: Ingestion of several grams of aspirin or other salicylate-containing products.

Epidem: Deliberate suicide attempt is the most common cause of toxic ingestions. Chronic salicylate toxicity is now rare.

Pathophys: Initially, toxic ingestions of salicylates produce respiratory alkalosis by direct stimulation of the CNS respiratory center. As the poisoning progresses, salicylates disrupt oxidative phosphorylation and several steps involved in carbohydrate metabolism, leading to accumulation of organic acids and profound metabolic acidosis. As the illness progresses, volume depletion and superimposed lactic acidosis are common. Brain hypoglycemia, even when the serum glucose is normal, is an important phenomenon seen in salicylate poisoning.

Sx: Nausea, vomiting, tinnitus, dizziness.

Si: Elevated body temperature and volume depletion due to vomiting can be seen. Neurological manifestations may progress from confusion to coma in a matter of hours.

Crs: Can be fatal if untreated, although the mortality with acute overdose is less than 10%. Mortality may be higher with chronic overdose.

Cmplc: Death.

Lab: Multiple electrolyte abnormalities will be present along with anion gap metabolic acidosis. Direct determination of the serum salicylate level is available at most labs. The Done nomogram can be used to estimate the severity of poisoning when the time of the ingestion is known. Caution should be used as enterically coated and sustained release preparations will be absorbed slower and will reach toxic levels later.

Rx: Salicylate poisoning treatment is aimed at reducing the cerebral tissue salicylate concentration. Patients with salicylate poisoning can have CNS hypoglycemia even when serum glucose is normal; therefore, supplemental glucose should be provided if mental status changes are present (J Clin Invest 1970;49:2139). Plasma alkalinization should be initiated to achieve an arterial pH of 7.45–7.55. Patients with aspirin poisoning may present with a high arterial pH, but it should not preclude administration of sodium bicarbonate. Frequent ABG monitoring and serum salicylate level measurements are needed to prevent excessive alkalemia (pH > 7.6) and to monitor treatment efficacy. Peak salicylate concentration can occur many hours after the ingestion, especially in cases of bezoar formation and intoxication with enterically coated preparations (Postgrad Med J 1991;89:61).

Alkalinization of urine to a pH of 8.0, while difficult to achieve, is desirable and will more than quadruple the rate of salicylate excretion compared to a urine pH of 6.5. Do *not* use acetazolamide to alkalinize the urine of the salicylate-poisoned patient, as it will increase tissue levels of salicylate. Endotracheal intubation requires extreme caution in this setting, as it will often be impossible to provide the very high minute ventilation required for these patients using a mechanical ventilator. Hemodialysis is indicated for patients with mental status changes, pulmonary or cerebral edema, or a very high serum salicylate concentration (> 80 mg/dL) (Kidney Int 1988;33:735, Clin Nephrol 1998;50:178).

Metabolic Acidosis due to Renal Failure

Cause: CKD or AKI

Epidem: The prevalence of this condition increases with increasing severity of CKD or duration of AKI.

Pathophys: Kidney failure causes acidosis through retention of hydrogen along with sulfate, urate, and phosphate anions.

Sx/Si: Metabolic acidosis due to CKD is usually asymptomatic. Hyperpnea and subjective shortness of breath may be present.

Crs: Acidosis in CKD is usually mild.

Cmplc: Chronic metabolic acidosis may exacerbate renal bone disease, uremic malnutrition, and progression of CKD.

Lab: ABG and serum electrolytes.

Rx: CKD patients should be treated with alkali to maintain a serum bicarbonate concentration above 22 mEq/L per KDOQI guideline recommendations. Alkali therapy may prevent loss of skeletal muscle (Kidney Int 1991;40:779) and may have beneficial effects on renal osteodystrophy (Kidney Int 1995;47:1816).

Normal Anion Gap Metabolic Acidosis (Hyperchloremic Acidosis)

Cause: Gastrointestinal losses of bicarbonate due to diarrhea, laxative abuse, ureterosigmoidostomy, and ileal conduit (usually in cases of ostomy stenosis); renal bicarbonate losses or renal dysfunction in renal tubular acidosis, some forms of renal failure, and administration of certain types of hyperalimentation fluids

Pathophys: All gastrointestinal secretions below the stomach are alkaline. Loss of these secretions due to diarrhea, diversion, tube drainage, or vomiting of small bowel contents will lead to metabolic acidosis. Some patients who abuse laxatives can present with a metabolic alkalosis in spite of diarrhea (poorly understood phenomenon). Ureteral diversion into the sigmoid colon leads to reabsorption of chloride and secretion of bicarbonate. Reabsorption of ammonium in the colon, with subsequent conversion to ammonia in the liver, also contributes to acidosis. Buffering of acid in bone can lead to loss of bone calcium with resulting osteomalacia and hypercalciuria with kidney stones (Am J Med 1997;102:477). Ileal conduit urinary diversion is less likely to have these effects due to decreased contact time between the urine and the ileal mucosa, because the urine drains rapidly into the ostomy bag (Lancet 1999;353:1813).

RTA is a rare disorder in which metabolic acidosis develops due to reduced urinary H^+ excretion. The diagnosis of RTA is reserved for patients with normal or near normal kidney function. It is impossible to diagnose RTA in severe renal failure where acidosis must be attributed to the inability to excrete acid due to low GFR.

Type 1 (distal) RTA is characterized by impaired distal urinary acidification and can be idiopathic, inherited, or more commonly, associated with autoimmune disease, especially Sjögren's syndrome in adults. Treatment with ifosfamide, amphotericin B, or exposure to toluene (glue sniffing) can result in a similar presentation (see Table 2.1 for a complete list of causes of type 1 RTA). Potassium wasting is usually present, and serum potassium is usually very low. In some cases, hypercalciuria, nephrolithiasis, and nephrocalcinosis can be seen.

Table 2.1   Causes of Renal Tubular Acidosis

Type 1 RTA (distal)

Idiopathic
Drug Induced
   Amphotericin B
   Ifosfamide
Toxin
   Toluene (glue sniffing)
Hematological Disorders
   Multiple myeloma
Hereditary
Idiopathic

Table 2.1   Causes of Renal Tubular Acidosis (continued)

Ehlers-Danlos syndrome
Marfan's syndrome
Wilson's disease
Hereditary eliptocytosis
Autoimmune Diseases
  Systemic lupus erythematosus
  Sjögren's syndrome
  Primary biliary cirrhosis
  Hypergammaglobulenemia
Disorders with Nephrocalcinosis
  Primary hyperparathyroidism
  Hypercalciuria
  Vitamin D intoxication

Type 2 RTA (proximal)

Idiopathic
Drugs
  Ifosfamide
  Acetozolomide
Toxins
  Lead
  Mercury
  Cadmium
Hematological disorders
  Multiple myeloma
  Amyloidosis
  Vitamin D deficiency with hypocalcemia
Hereditary
  Cystinosis
  Wilson's disease
  Glycogen storage diseases
  Lowe's syndrome
  Hereditary fructose intolerance
  Galactosemia

Type 2 (proximal) RTA is due to reduced proximal bicarbonate reabsorption. Use of acetazolamide and multiple myeloma are the most common causes of this condition (see Table 2.1 for a complete list of causes of type 2 RTA). Because bicarbonate is reabsorbed in the distal nephron, these patients tend to have only a moderate acidosis with serum bicarbonate, usually maintained between 14 and 20 mEq/L. The severity of hypokalemia is variable. This disorder can be accompanied by diffuse proximal tubular dysfunction (Fanconi syndrome) (Kidney Int 1981;20:705).

Type 3 RTA is a term that is no longer in use. It previously described a disorder seen in infants that is currently classified as a subtype of type 1 RTA.

Type 4 RTA is a disorder of aldosterone deficiency that is usually seen in diabetic patients with mild renal impairment. Hyperkalemia is the most prominent feature of type 4 RTA. Dx and rx of type 4 RTA are described in Chapter 1.4.

Crs: In cases of mild acidosis due to diarrhea, the acidosis will resolve spontaneously when the gastrointestinal illness is controlled. This is especially true for patients with normal renal function. Patients with ileal conduits who become acidotic should be investigated for the presence of ileal conduit obstruction with a loopogram.

Patients with type 1 RTA will be either asymptomatic or will have symptoms due to severe hypokalemia (muscle weakness, polyuria, polydipsia) or symptomatic kidney stones. Patients with type 2 RTA develop rickets as children and osteopenia as adults (N Engl J Med 1982;307:217).

Lab: ABG, electrolytes, BUN, Cr, Mg, Ca, urine pH, urine Na, K, Cl, diarrhea workup.

If the diagnosis is not clear from hx, blood tests, and urine pH, then urine anion gap should be calculated.

$$\text{Urine AG} = \text{urine NA} + \text{urine K} - \text{urine Cl}$$

Urine AG will be negative in most patients with diarrhea or other gastrointestinal losses but will be positive in type 1 RTA, renal failure, and type 4 RTA (hypoaldosteronism). Urine AG is especially useful in patients with hypokalemia caused by diarrhea or toluene exposure who may have relatively high urine pH, which may suggest a type 1 RTA. However, an appropriately negative AG, especially with an hx of diarrhea, will lead to a correct dx. Urine AG cannot be used in volume-depleted patients (N Engl J Med 1988;318:594).

To differentiate type 2 from type 1 RTA, serum bicarbonate should be raised with a bicarbonate infusion followed by the measurement of urine pH and fractional excretion of bicarbonate. In type 2 RTA, urine pH will rise dramatically, and the fractional excretion of bicarbonate will rise to 15%–20%. These parameters will usually remain unchanged in type 1 RTA.

$$\text{FE HCO}_3^- = (\text{urine HCO}_3 \times \text{serum Cr}) / (\text{serum HCO}_3 \times \text{urine Cr}) \times 100\%$$

Rx: Treatment of metabolic acidosis due to diarrhea and other forms of gastrointestinal bicarbonate loss is directed at control of gastrointestinal bicarbonate loss. Mild acidosis will correct spontaneously and does not require alkali administration. If acidosis is severe, bicarbonate replacement can be given provided that hypokalemia and hypocalcemia have been treated because administration of bicarbonate will exacerbate those conditions. Patients with ureterosigmoidostomy can be treated with sodium bicarbonate or sodium citrate to prevent bone loss and kidney stones. If acidosis develops in a patient with an ileal conduit, an evaluation for conduit obstruction should be undertaken. Correction of conduit problems will minimize urine to conduit contact time and improve the acidosis. Type 1 and type 2 RTA are treated with sodium bicarbonate or sodium citrate. In type 1 RTA, correction of acidosis will correct potassium wasting and improve hypokalemia. Type 2 RTA can be very difficult to treat as the kidneys can rapidly waste administered bicarbonate, and large doses may be needed. In pediatric disease, correction of acidosis is needed in order to allow for normal growth (Kidney Int 1981;20:799). Treatment of type 4 RTA is directed mostly at correction of hyperkalemia. Neither sodium bicarbonate nor sodium citrate is usually administered because type 4 RTA patients tend to have mild renal dysfunction, and administration of alkali can exacerbate their edema and hypertension.

2.4   Metabolic Alkalosis

(J Nephrol 2006;19 Suppl 9:S86; Rose BD, Post TW, Clinical Physiology of Acid-Base and Electrolyte Disorders, New York; McGraw-Hill, 2001)

Cause: Metabolic alkalosis usually occurs due to diuretic therapy and loss of gastric secretions through vomiting and nasogastric tube suction. Less common causes include primary mineralocorticoid excess (adrenal adenoma or hyperplasia, renin-secreting kidney tumor, ACTH-secreting pituitary tumor, Cushing's disease, and glucocorticoid-remediable hyperaldosteronism); apparent mineralocorticoid excess (licorice ingestion, Liddle's syndrome, and 11 β-hydroxysteroid dehydrogenase deficiency); severe hypokalemia; milk alkali syndrome; diarrhea due to villous adenoma and laxative abuse; Bartter's and Gitelman's syndromes; volume depletion due to sweat losses in cystic fibrosis; and rapid correction of chronic respiratory acidosis by mechanical ventilation (posthypercapnic alkalosis).

Pathophys: Loss of H^+ in gastrointestinal secretions or urine leads to generation of equal number of mEq of extracellular HCO_3^-. Loss of bicarbonate-free fluids via urinary or gastrointestinal tract or as sweat will lead to "contraction" of the extracellular fluid around a fixed amount of extracellular HCO_3^- and generation of contraction alkalosis (Ann Intern Med 1965;62:979). Under usual circumstances, renal excretion of bicarbonate will lead to rapid correction of metabolic alkalosis unless factors that interfere with the excretion of bicarbonate are present. Volume depletion, chloride depletion, and hypokalemia will all prevent reabsorption of bicarbonate at multiple nephron segments and will often work in concert to allow for maintenance of metabolic alkalosis (Kidney Int 1984;25:357).

Sx: Metabolic alkalosis itself is usually asymptomatic. Since volume depletion is frequently present, patients may report symptoms of hypovolemia such as weakness, dizziness, and cramps. Neurological abnormalities seen in posthypercapnic alkalosis are due to sudden reduction in pCO_2 and not to high serum HCO_3 (JAMA 1964;189:993).

Si: Patients with metabolic alkalosis will often exhibit signs of volume depletion such as poor skin turgor and postural hypotension. In cases of self-induced vomiting, physical findings common in bulimia (calluses on the dorsum of the hand, poor dentition, salivary gland swelling) will be present (Am Fam Physician 2003;67:297).

Crs: After metabolic alkalosis develops, it will persist until the factor responsible for the maintenance of alkalosis, such as volume depletion or hypokalemia, resolves. In patients with hypovolemia due to gastrointestinal or renal fluid losses, correction of sodium chloride deficit will lead to rapid correction of alkalosis. Potassium replacement will have a similar effect in profoundly hypokalemic patients. In patients with edematous states, such as CHF or cirrhosis, who require diuretics chronically for the control of edema, alkalosis may be persistent.

ACID-BASE DISORDERS

Cmplc: Since hypokalemia is often present in patients with heart disease who are alkalemic due to diuretics, these same patients are at risk of cardiac arrhythmias (Am J Cardiol 1990;65:4E).

Lab: Elevated serum bicarbonate can be present in chronic respiratory acidosis or metabolic alkalosis. Measurement of the arterial pH can help differentiate these disorders. Once metabolic acidosis is confirmed, measure serum and urine electrolytes. In metabolic alkalosis, urine sodium is not a reliable measure of volume status. The need for increased sodium bicarbonate excretion will lead to high urine sodium even when hypovolemia is present. In this situation, low urine Cl (< 25 mEq/L) will be a better indicator of the volume depletion that occurs with vomiting. In patients with mineralocorticoid excess, apparent mineralocorticoid excess, and alkali ingestion, urine chloride will usually be high (> 40 mEq/L).

In hypertensive patients with alkalosis, measurement of serum renin and aldosterone levels may lead to the diagnosis of mineralocorticoid excess. If hypertension and high urine chloride are present but aldosterone is not elevated, syndromes of apparent mineralocorticoid excess should be suspected.

Rx: Normal saline and potassium repletion will correct posthypercapnic alkalosis and metabolic alkalosis due to vomiting, NG tube suction, and diuretics.

Edematous patients with heart failure or cirrhosis who develop metabolic alkalosis on diuretic therapy should not be treated with saline to avoid worsening edema. Diuretics should be minimized whenever possible, and hypokalemia should be corrected. The carbonic anhydrase inhibitor acetazolamide will help control the edema and correct metabolic acidosis by increasing renal excretion of bicarbonate. While the administration of hydrochloric acid in severe metabolic alkalosis has been described (Lancet 1983;1:953), it is usually not needed in routine practice because alkalosis is usually well tolerated.

Unilateral aldosterone-secreting tumors usually require surgical removal but can sometimes be treated medically in patients who are poor surgical candidates. Primary hyperaldosteronism can be treated with spironolactone or eplerenone (more expensive than spironolactone but has fewer side effects). Surgical treatment is less effective for adrenal hyperplasia than for unilateral tumors (Endocrinology 2003;144:2208). The very rare renin-secreting kidney tumors are treated surgically (J Urol 1995;153:1781). Glucocorticoid-remediable hyperaldosteronism is treated with dexamethazone (Cardiol Rev 2004;12:44). Liddle's syndrome will respond to triamterene or amiloride, which directly closes the mutant sodium channel in the collecting tubule (N Engl J Med 1994;330:178).

2.5 Respiratory Acidosis

(Rose BD, Post TW, Clinical Physiology of Acid-Base and Electrolyte Disorders, New York; McGraw-Hill, 2001)

Cause: Hypercapnia (increase of pCO_2) can occur due to lung disorders resulting in impaired gas exchange; airway obstruction, which can be chronic (such as in COPD), or acute (such as in aspiration and sleep apnea); inhibition of the respiratory center in the CNS by depressant drugs; obesity hypoventilation; and muscle and neurological disorders that result in respiratory muscle weakness.

Pathophys: Even a minor elevation in arterial pCO_2 quickly stimulates respiration in normal subjects. A drop in arterial pO_2 also stimulates respiration, although this occurs with a relatively large decrease in pO_2 to 60 mm Hg. Because CO_2 diffuses across the alveolar membranes 20 times faster than oxygen, individuals who experience an acute respiratory disorder while breathing room air will develop hypoxemia before they develop hypercapnia.

Individuals with chronic respiratory acidosis are less sensitive to CO_2-induced increase in ventilation. In these patients, hypoxemia acts as the primary ventilatory stimulus.

Sx: While dyspnea is the common symptom of respiratory disorders, acute respiratory acidosis can result is a variety of CNS symptoms, such as anxiety, restlessness, headaches, delirium, and diminished level of arousal (CO_2 narcosis). Patients with chronic respiratory acidosis will frequently have chronic dyspnea and wheezing related to their chronic lung disease, such as asthma or COPD. Lung disorders leading to pulmonary hypertension and right heart failure will lead to edema. Patients with sleep apnea will have daytime somnolence, snoring, headaches, and fatigue.

Si: Abnormal lung exam or evidence of right heart failure can be present.

Crs: Severe acute respiratory acidosis can be rapidly fatal unless steps to restore ventilation, such as administration of antidote (naloxone, flumazenil) to patients who have lost their respiratory drive due to a CNS depressant overdose (narcotics or benzodiazepines) or mechanical ventilations for patients with other lung disorders, are instituted. Chronic respiratory acidosis in individuals with chronic lung disease is often a chronic condition with stable renal compensation.

Cmplc: Acute cases of CO_2 narcosis can lead to death. Chronic respiratory acidosis can have a prolonged course with exacerbations.

Lab: ABG, serum electrolytes

Rx: Use invasive or noninvasive mechanical ventilation for severe acute respiratory acidosis, especially when associated with hypoxemia. Use antidotes for respiratory depressants, when possible. Sodium bicarbonate administration is rarely indicated and should be viewed as the treatment of last resort to maintain a safe pH when adequate ventilation cannot be achieved.

Treatment of chronic respiratory acidosis centers on avoidance of hypoxemia without administration of excessive oxygen, which can suppress ventilation along with treatment of the underlying lung disease. Administration of sodium bicarbonate is not a standard part of therapy of respiratory acidosis and should be reserved only for special situations where the need to maintain an acceptable arterial pH when the pCO_2 cannot be corrected due to severe ventilation problems.

2.6 Respiratory Alkalosis

(Rose BD, Post TW, Clinical Physiology of Acid-Base and Electrolyte Disorders, New York; McGraw-Hill, 2001)

Cause: Hyperventilation resulting in hypocapnia and elevation of the arterial pH. This can be caused by hypoxemia, severe anemia, pain, sepsis, or anxiety. Direct stimulation of the respiratory center within the CNS can occur due to salicylates, progesterone, toxins retained in liver failure, or psychiatric disease. Respiratory alkalosis can occur when mechanical ventilation is prescribed with excessive minute ventilation.

Pathophys: Just minutes after the onset of excessive ventilation, intracellular hydrogen ions move into the extracellular space where they react with bicarbonate ions, producing a drop in serum bicarbonate. For each 10 mm Hg drop in arterial pCO_2, bicarbonate will acutely decline by 2 mEq/L.

If the respiratory alkalosis becomes chronic after being present for several days, renal excretion of bicarbonate will increase, and serum bicarbonate will drop by 4 mEq/L for each 10 mm Hg drop in arterial pCO_2.

Sx/Si: Nervous system irritability with dizziness, lightheadedness, changes of mental status, and paresthesias, cramps, and carpopedal spasm. A variety of arrhythmias can also occur.

ACID-BASE DISORDERS

Crs: Respiratory alkalosis will usually resolve spontaneously when the precipitating factor is corrected or when mechanical ventilation is adjusted.

Cmplc: Usually related to underlying cause

Lab: ABG, serum electrolytes

Rx: Treatment of underlying cause. In mechanically ventilated patients, minute ventilation can be reduced by reducing respiratory rate or tidal volume.

Chapter 3

Acute Kidney Injury

(N Engl J Med 1996;334:1448)

Introduction: Acute kidney injury (AKI) is a term that describes several syndromes characterized by a sudden (hours to weeks) decline in kidney function. Prior to the onset of AKI, either normal GFR or chronically impaired renal function may be present. The latter condition is commonly referred to as "acute on chronic" kidney disease. The decline in GFR is usually recognized as either an increase in BUN and Cr or a sudden decline in urine output. There is no universally agreed upon definition of AKI; however, a rise in Cr by 0.5 mg/dL in patients with normal renal function and by 1.0 mg/dL in individuals with pre-existing kidney disease has recently been used as a research definition (Kidney Int 2004;66:1613).

Traditional classification of AKI syndromes into prerenal AKI, intrinsic renal AKI, and obstruction (postrenal AKI) provides a useful framework for approaching this condition in the clinical setting.

3.1 Approach to a Patient with Acute Kidney Injury

(N Engl J Med 1996;334:1448)

Diagnosis: In most cases, the cause of AKI (formerly called acute renal failure) is readily apparent from the clinical situation. The following are the issues that should be considered in the cases of AKI, where the cause may not be readily apparent:

- When AKI does not present in the hospital, a patient with azotemia may actually be suffering from chronic kidney disease. A kidney ultrasound that demonstrates small echogenic kidneys will help confirm the presence of CKD as opposed to AKI. Bland urinary sediment will further confirm this finding.
- Acute on chronic renal failure is common and requires knowledge of the prior level of kidney function for determination of severity.
- A history and physical will suggest the cause of AKI in most cases.
- Recent medical interventions, such as new medications, iv contrast studies, or procedures, are often associated with deterioration of renal function.
- Prerenal azotemia will be seen in patients who are truly dehydrated, with a history of volume depletion, and in 3 edematous conditions: CHF, cirrhosis, and the nephrotic syndrome.
- Patients with true volume depletion who are suspected of having prerenal azotemia should have prompt recovery of renal function after resuscitation. Failure to improve renal function immediately upon the correction of effective circulating volume suggests another cause of AKI.
- NSAIDs, ACEIs, and ARBs will predispose to prerenal azotemia and possibly further ischemic renal injury.
- Calcineurin inhibitors, cyclosporine, and tacrolimus can cause both hemodynamically mediated AKI, particularly at toxic levels, and CKD with prolonged administration.
- Urinalysis is critical for the workup of intrarenal AKI.
- Proteinuria, hematuria, and renal failure suggest a diagnosis of RPGN, where a prompt diagnosis may be required for the optimum outcome.
- In cases of ATN, one must consider ATN due to drugs and toxins, along with ischemic ATN.
- Myeloma kidney (cast nephropathy) should be considered in elderly individuals. Any renal hypoperfusion event may reduce

renal tubular flow and set off cast precipitation in a patient with preexisting myeloma.

- Sepsis is a risk factor for ATN even in the absence of hypotension, as inflammation can cause renal tubular injury directly.
- Iodinated iv contrast-induced ATN will have a rapid onset (hours to days). Deterioration of renal function weeks after an endovascular procedure suggests a diagnosis of cholesterol embolization.
- Production of urine does not exclude urinary tract obstruction.
- Complete obstruction of one kidney in a previously healthy individual should not produce a loss of more than 50% of kidney function unless another kidney disease is present in the kidney that is not obstructed.
- Complete cessation of urine output has a relatively narrow differential diagnosis of complete obstruction of the urinary tract, very severe ATN, type 1 hepatorenal syndrome or a vascular catastrophe with loss of circulation to both kidneys.

Treatment: The therapeutic approach to an AKI patient varies widely depending on the clinical setting. This section is intended to serve as a general guideline for approaching a patient with acute kidney injury.

- Obstruction of the urinary tract should be relieved as soon as possible.
- The choice of procedure for relieving the obstruction will depend on the location of the obstruction and will be discussed below.
- Nephrotoxic drugs as well as medications that interfere with glomerular perfusion, such as NSAIDs, ACEIs, ARBs, and in some cases diuretics, should be discontinued.
- Restoration of adequate circulating volume is often a critical step in the management of prerenal and intrarenal AKI. This critical step should receive adequate attention, particularly in sepsis, postsurgery, pancreatitis, and myoglobinuria.

- While the choice of iv fluid for resuscitation of hypovolemic patients will continue to be a subject of controversy, saline is still the safest and most effective option. In particular, the use of albumin was not demonstrated to be superior in a large trial (N Engl J Med 2004;350:2247). The only population in which albumin may be useful is patients with cirrhosis; albumin may have a role in the management or prevention of hepato-renal syndrome (Clin Liver Dis 2006;10:371; N Engl J Med 1999;341:403).
- While only a limited amount of information is available regarding the renal outcomes of early intensive, goal directed, protocol guided therapy of patients with septic shock, this therapy clearly improves the overall survival. The emphasis on the measurement of the CVP and reaching predetermined MAP and urine output goals has improved mortality and should be encouraged (N Engl J Med 2001;345:1368; Shock 2006;26:551).
- While the use of ionotropic agents (pressors) is frequently necessary for the maintenance of perfusion in AKI, there is no data that any of these agents (particularly dopamine) improve outcomes in AKI. Therefore, the use of dopamine for the treatment of AKI in the absence of another indication should be discouraged.
- The use of loop diuretics in patients with AKI in general and in those who are critically ill in particular should be discouraged as there is *no* evidence that they improve outcomes (JAMA 2002;288:2547). There may be compelling reasons to use diuretics for pulmonary edema, volume overload, hyperkalemia, and hypercalcemia.
- Even with meticulous attention to resuscitation and overall management of patients with AKI, some patients will require dialysis or another form of RRT.
- It is important to remember that thrice weekly intermittent hemodialysis used to treat stable outpatients with ESRD is

likely not the ideal therapy for hospitalized patients with AKI. There are substantial differences in the metabolism and fluid management of acutely ill patients when compared to ESRD patients that may require significant customization of the RRT prescription and schedule.

- Volume overload, hyperkalemia, uremic pericarditis, uremic encephalopathy, and severe acidosis that are not manageable with diuretics or other medical therapies constitute absolute indications for RRT.

- There is substantial variation in the timing of initiation of RRT in critically ill patients with AKI due to lack of evidence regarding the optimal timing of RRT initiation. While BUN over 100 mg/dL was previously considered to be an appropriate marker for initiation of RRT, there is emerging evidence that earlier initiation of RRT may be appropriate (Clin J Am Soc Nephrol 2006;1:903).

- RRT modality for critically ill patients with AKI is also a subject of controversy. While continuous therapies such as SCUF, CVVH, CVVHD, and CVVHDF are appealing because they are believed to be better hemodynamically tolerated, there is controversy as to whether they lead to better outcomes. These treatments require highly specialized equipment, continuous anticoagulation, and specially prepared dialysate and/or replacement solutions; therefore, these methodologies involve considerable technical challenges that introduce additional risks when compared to intermittent HD (Nat Clin Pract Nephrol 2007;3:118).

    - SCUF is a method of slow fluid removal by ultrafiltration only. SCUF may be useful in hypotensive patients with fluid overload. This approach results in very minimal solute removal and is not appropriate for patients with severe uremia or electrolyte or acid-base disorders. SCUF has many technical similarities to the ultrafiltration approach to the treatment of CHF described in Chapter 3.5. Traditionally the term SCUF is reserved for a technique applied to unstable patients. Unlike the new specialized equipment described in Chapter 3.5, traditional equipment capable of performing SCUF requires continuous anticoagulation.

- CVVH involves high ultrafiltration rates of at least 1 L/hr. CVVH is a convective treatment where small and medium solute is removed by solvent drag as opposed to diffusion. Because a large amount of ultrafiltrate is removed, replacement fluid must be administered. Manipulating the electrolyte composition of the replacement fluid allows for correction of electrolyte disorders. Replacing a smaller amount of fluid than the amount of ultrafiltrate removed allows one to achieve a prescribed fluid removal.

- CVVHD is similar to conventional HD, but it utilizes much slower rates of blood and dialysate flow, which in theory should allow for avoidance of hemodynamic instability due to rapid solute removal. CVVHD is preferred over CVVH in situations where rapid removal of small solutes is required. Diffusive clearance of small solutes such as potassium is higher than their convective clearance, so CVVHD is preferred for the treatment of unstable patients with severe hyperkalemia or acidosis.

- CVVHDF is a combination of CVVH and CVVHD, which occur simultaneously. This modality combines the higher clearance of medium-size solutes by convection with the high clearance of small molecules by diffusion. This technique is the most complicated of all continuous therapies.

- While the use of continuous techniques in critically ill patients is attractive due to a perception that they are better hemodynamically tolerated, there is some evidence that they may not offer a survival advantage to critically ill patients with AKI, particularly when compared to intermittent dialysis that utilizes many newer technologies (Am J Kidney Dis 2002;40:875; Clin J Am Soc Nephrol 2007;2:385).

- New therapies, such as SLEDD, will further complicate the issues related to selection of RRT modality for the critically ill patient.

3.2   Prerenal Azotemia

Introduction: Prerenal azotemia usually develops in the context of another illness or treatment of illness. Since medications that alter glomerular hemodynamics frequently contribute to and sometimes cause this condition, common medication-induced azotemia scenarios will be discussed along with hemodynamically induced prerenal azotemia.

Hemodynamically Induced Prerenal Azotemia

Cause: Hemodynamic conditions that lead to renal hypoperfusion.

- Any cause of true intravascular volume depletion, such as:
  - Vomiting or diarrhea
  - Renal fluid losses due to diuretic therapy
  - Blood loss
  - Skin losses due to burns
  - "Third spacing" of fluid due to sepsis or pancreatitis
- Effective circulating volume depletion due to: CHF, cirrhosis, or nephrotic syndrome.
- Intrarenal vasoconstriction due to: NSAIDs, cyclosporine, tacrolimus; hypercalcemia.
- Efferent arteriole vasodilatation due to: ACEIs and ARBs (particularly in volume depleted subjects).

Epidem: Data on epidemiology of AKI is difficult to interpret since most studies are targeted at hospitalized patients. Among hospitalized patients in a developed country, prerenal azotemia is the second most common cause of AKI after ATN (Kidney Int 1996;50:811). Epidemiology of AKI is quite different in the

ACUTE KIDNEY INJURY

developing world where volume depletion due to diarrhea and hemolysis due to malaria cause many cases of AKI.

Pathophys: True hypovolemia or effective circulating volume depletion leads to decreased renal perfusion, which results in the reduction in GFR without injury to the tubular cells. Often agents that interfere with glomerular autoregulation, such as NSAIDs, ACEIs, or ARBs, are contributing.

Sx: Fatigue, nausea (especially upon awakening), vomiting, loss of appetite, shortness of breath, pruritis, confusion, and changes of mental status

Si: In cases of dehydration, hypotension or orthostatic hypotension, poor skin turgor, and dry mucous membranes will be present. In cases of effective circulating volume depletion such as CHF, cirrhosis or nephrosis, signs of volume overload such as edema and rales will be present.

Crs: In situations where true intravascular volume depletion is present (vomiting, diarrhea, bleeding), BUN and Cr will return to normal as soon as hypovolemia is corrected. In conditions such as CHF and cirrhosis, the course of prerenal azotemia will reflect the state of the underlying condition.

Cmplc: Progression to ATN if timely resuscitation does not occur. Complications of renal failure such as hyperkalemia, anemia, metabolic acidosis, hyponatremia, and pericarditis may occur. Complications can result from accumulation of routine medications (such as hypoglycemia due to accumulation of sulfonylureas or insulin, bradycardia and hypotension due to accumulation of water-soluble beta-blockers, and complications due to accumulation of antibiotics and others).

Lab: BUN, Cr, CBC, electrolytes, urinalysis

Urine sodium will be less than 10 mmol/L. Urine specific gravity will be greater than 1.020 in prerenal azotemia. Urine sodium is typically greater than 20 mmol/L and urine specific gravity is 1.010–1.020 in intrinsic renal conditions. Fractional excretion of sodium will be < 1% in prerenal azotemia as opposed to > 1% in ATN.

$$\text{Fractional excretion Na} = (U_{Na}/P_{Na}) / (U_{cr}/P_{cr})$$

BUN to Cr ratio of greater than 20 is typically seen in prerenal azotemia, but it can also be seen in a variety of other conditions such as urinary tract obstruction, high protein intake, gastrointestinal bleeding, and corticosteroid therapy. In patients receiving diuretics, fractional excretion of urea can be calculated in a manner similar to fractional excretion of sodium.

$$\text{Fractional excretion Urea} = (U_{BUN}/P_{BUN}) / (U_{cr}/P_{cr})$$

Fractional excretion of urea of ≤ 35% may be a more specific index than fractional excretion of sodium for the diagnosis of prerenal azotemia as opposed to ATN, especially in patients receiving diuretics (Kidney Int 2002;62:2223).

Xray: Renal ultrasound may help exclude obstruction as a possible explanation for AKI.

Rx: In cases of true intravascular volume depletion, volume expansion with normal saline, lactated ringers solution, or oral rehydration should lead to prompt resolution of renal failure as soon as the volume deficit is corrected. If, after adequate resuscitation, renal function remains impaired, another cause of AKI must be present. In cases of effective circulating volume depletion such as in advanced CHF or cirrhosis, optimization of the underlying condition, if possible, may lead to improvement in renal function.

3.3 ACEI- and ARB-Induced Prerenal Azotemia

(Am Heart J 1999;138:849)

Cause: Interference with renin-angiotensin system, particularly in subjects with volume depletion, diuretic therapy, heart failure, hypotension, or renovascular disease

Epidem: Older subjects, particularly with CHF or CKD, and those concurrently on NSAIDs. In the SOLVD trial (Studies of Left Ventricular Dysfunction), AKI was 33% more likely in subjects receiving enalapril.

Pathophys: Inability to maintain intraglomerular pressure with resulting decline in GFR due to blockade of the renin-angiotensin system controlled constriction of the efferent arteriole.

Sx: Symptoms of prerenal azotemia as described in the above hemodynamic prerenal azotemia section.

Si: Possibly hypotension

Crs: Many patients will experience stable, predictable, and acceptable decline in GFR that will allow for continued treatment. If a compelling indication for ACEI or ARB therapy exists, treatment can usually be continued with close monitoring of renal function (N Engl J Med 2006;354:131). Alternatively, an unacceptable decline in GFR may occur.

Cmplc: Progression to ATN, hyperkalemia

Lab: BUN, Cr, electrolytes, CBC

Rx: Acceptable decline in GFR with ACEI and ARB use should be monitored while the rx is continued. It has been suggested that these agents be discontinued if serum Cr rises by more than 30% from the baseline value. Patients, particularly those simultaneously treated with diuretics, should be advised to discontinue ACEI or ARB if they develop an illness that is likely to lead to volume depletion (gastrointestinal conditions with vomiting or diarrhea) or hypotension.

All patients should undergo measurement of baseline renal function and serum potassium before the initiation of therapy and 1 wk after starting the drug and after every dose increase.

3.4 NSAID-Induced Prerenal Azotemia and Acute Tubular Necrosis

(Am J Kidney Dis 1996;28:S56)

Cause: Both nonselective and selective COX-2 inhibitors interfere with the synthesis of vasodilating prostaglandins and afferent artery vasoconstriction. This can, in turn, lead to prerenal azotemia.

Epidem: Individuals with CHF, preexisting CKD, atherosclerotic renovascular disease and the elderly are especially at risk. Use of high-dose NSAIDs can more than double the risk of AKI in the elderly, including AKI requiring hospitalization (Am J Epidemiol 2000;151:488).

Pathophys: Afferent arteriole vasoconstriction due to NSAIDs' interference with vasodilatory prostaglandins

Sx: Symptoms of prerenal azotemia as described in the above hemodynamic prerenal azotemia section

Si: Hypertension, edema, pulmonary edema

Crs: May progress to ATN in the presence of confounding factors such as CHF. In individuals with preexisting CKD, failure to recover from AKI and progression of CKD may occur.

Cmplc: Any complication of renal failure can occur. Hypertension, volume overload, and hyperkalemia are particularly common in this setting.

Lab: BUN, Cr, electrolytes, CBC

Rx: Discontinuation of the offending agent and rx of complications

ACUTE KIDNEY INJURY

3.5   Intrinsic Causes of AKI

(N Engl J Med 1996;334:1448)

Introduction: Intrarenal causes of AKI are traditionally classified
according to the location of the involved compartment inside the
kidney as shown in Table 3.1. ATN is by far the most common
cause of intrinsic AKI, and it will be discussed first. While each
condition is discussed separately in this section, they often coexist, particularly in severely ill hospitalized patients.

Table 3.1   Causes of Intrarenal Acute Kidney Injury

Acute Tubular Necrosis

Due to ischemia
  Shock
      Hypovolemic
      Septic
      Cardiogenic
  Surgery
      Hypotension
      Renal artery clamp
      Cardiopulmonary bypass
  Multifactorial
      Combination of the following
      Volume depletion
      Diuretics
      ACEI or ARB
      NSAIDs
      Other nephrotoxins
Due to toxins
  Drugs
      Aminoglycoside antibiotics
      Cisplatinum
      Amphotericin B
  Iodinated IV contrast
  Toxins
      Intravascular hemolysis

Table 3.1   Causes of Intrarenal Acute Kidney Injury (continued)

Rhabdomyolysis
Myeloma protein

Hepatorenal Syndrome

Acute Interstitial Nephritis

Drugs
  Antibiotics
  NSAIDs
  Furosemide
  Acyclovir crystals
  Indinavir crystals
  Uric acid crystals
Infection
  Tuberculosis
  Bacterial
  Viral
Autoimmune
  SLE
  Sarcoidodosis
Malignant
  Multiple myeloma
  Infiltration by Lymphoma
  Infiltration by other tumors

Rapidly Progressive Glomerulonephritis

ANCA Vasculitis
SLE
Postinfectious GN
Poststreptococcal GN
Anti-GBM disease
IgA nephropathy and HSP

Vascular Disorders

Cholesterol embolization
TTP/HUS
Renal artery dissection
Renal vein thrombosis

3.6 Acute Tubular Necrosis

Ischemic ATN

Cause: Renal hypoperfusion resulting in tubular cell death. There is a continuum of damage that occurs as the result of renal hypoperfusion. As renal blood flow becomes impaired, prerenal azotemia develops; this will be promptly reversible if renal perfusion is restored. If hypoperfusion becomes more severe or prolonged, tubular cell injury and death will occur, and the tubular cells will require time to heal even after restoration of perfusion. While most cases of ATN are reversible, in especially severe cases irreversible cortical necrosis can occur.

Epidem: ATN is usually a complication of another illness when diagnosed in the hospital setting. ATN accounts for 85% of AKI episodes. Ischemic ATN is more common than toxin-induced ATN.

Pathophys: As renal ischemia progresses past the reversible stage of prerenal azotemia, renal epithelial and endothelial cell injury occurs, followed by global renal vasoconstriction.

Si: While urine output may be low, it is highly variable, and some patients can have very low GFR with a near normal urine output (nonoliguric AKI).

Sx: Many patients will have another severe illness, with its attendant symptoms. Symptoms of acute uremia include nausea (especially upon awakening), vomiting, poor appetite, lethargy, confusion, and shortness of breath.

Crs: The outcome of ischemic ATN is critically dependent on the outcome of the underlying illness causing it and the severity of other comorbidities. The mortality rate of patients with multisystem organ failure may approach 100% in especially severe cases of critical illness. While the development of AKI is related to the severity of the underlying illness, the development of AKI does dramatically increase the risk of death even when statistical adjustment for other comorbidities is made. This suggests that ATN alone increases mortality dramatically (Am J Med 1998;104:343). If the patient survives, renal function will be likely to recover with a good long-term outcome. Progression to cortical necrosis is rare. The need for chronic dialysis in patients whose renal function was normal prior to the onset of ATN is rare.

Cmplc: Hyperkalemia, metabolic acidosis, volume overload

Lab: Serum electrolytes, BUN, Cr, urinalysis

The classic finding of brown granular casts, also called muddy brown casts, is neither sensitive nor specific. In cases of ATN, urine sodium should not be low, and fractional excretion of sodium will be high. This will help differentiate ATN from prerenal azotemia.

$$\text{Fractional excretion Na} = (U_{Na}/P_{Na}) \,/\, (U_{cr}/P_{cr})$$

Fractional excretion of sodium will be > 1% in ATN as opposed to < 1% in prerenal azotemia.

Rx: There is no specific rx for prevention of progression to ATN once hemodynamic insult has progressed to cell injury. RRT will support the patient while the underlying illness is being treated until renal recovery occurs. There is no consensus on the timing of initiation of RRT in AKI. Traditional indications for AKI are hyperkalemia, volume overload resistant to diuretics, severe metabolic acidosis, pericarditis, and uremic encephalopathy.

3.7 Radiocontrast and Other Toxin-Induced Kidney Injury

Introduction: Major causes of toxin-induced ATN are shown in Table 3.1. Because there is a broad variety of endogenous and exogenous causes of drug-induced ATN, many of the more important causes will be described separately.

Radiocontrast Induced ATN

(N Engl J Med 2006;354:379)

Cause: Iodinated iv contrast

Epidem: Radiocontrast nephropathy is the third most common cause of hospital acquired AKI (Am J Kidney Dis 2002;39:930). The baseline level of kidney function is a critical determinant of risk for AKI. If kidney function is normal prior to the procedure, AKI is unlikely. Risk increases continuously as GFR decreases. Risk factors for the development of radiocontrast nephropathy are DM, age > 75, volume depletion before the procedure, CHF, cirrhosis, nephrotic syndrome, concomitant use of NSAIDs, hypotension, and the use of an aortic balloon pump. Administration of a high volume of contrast increases the risk of AKI.

Pathophys: Pathogenesis is poorly understood. Reactive oxygen species, medullary vasoconstriction, and changes in vasoactive mediators occur.

Sx: Low urine output and sx of uremia and volume overload

Crs: AKI is usually transient. Peak serum creatinine will occur 3 days post procedure, and full recovery of renal function is common by 10 days after the procedure. The need for dialysis is rare unless renal function is very poor prior to the procedure or if the patient is in the highest risk group (hypotension, volume depletion, aortic balloon pump, and high volume of contrast).

Cmplc: Contrast-induced AKI has been shown to be associated with an increased length of hospital stay, cardiac complications such as CHF, and increased mortality.

Lab: Serum electrolytes, BUN, Cr, urinalysis. (The classic finding of brown granular casts, also called muddy brown casts, is neither sensitive nor specific.)

Rx: Assessment of risk is the first step. If the risk of radiocontrast nephropathy is high, consider imaging without iv contrast or alternative imaging modalities. If no alternative exists, discontinuation of nephrotoxic agents, volume expansion, and use of the minimal required volume of low-osmolar or isoosmolar contrast should be undertaken.

Patients with stage 4 or 5 CKD need to be counseled regarding the possible need for dialysis after the procedure as well as the possibility of progression to ESRD. This situation requires a nephrology consultation and possible planning for dialysis. Several regimens for volume expansion with isotonic fluid have been proposed. Volume expansion with normal saline remains the cornerstone prophylactic rx for the prevention of radiocontrast nephropathy in high-risk patients. N-acetylcysteine (600 mg bid for 4 doses starting prior to the administration of contrast) is widely used due to its favorable safety profile, although its efficacy remains controversial. The following volume expansion protocols have been suggested based on the available data:

1. Intravenous normal (0.9%) saline at 1 ml/kg/hr for 24 hr beginning several hours prior to radiocontrast administration
2. Intravenous sodium bicarbonate 154 mEq/L at 3 ml/kg/hr prior to radiocontrast administration and then at 1 ml/kg/hr for 6 hr after radiocontrast administration. This regimen was proposed based on a single randomized trial in which it was shown to be superior to 0.9% saline (JAMA 2004;291:2328).

Aminoglycoside-Induced ATN

(Postgrad Med J 1996;100:83)

Cause: Aminoglycoside antibiotics (gentamicin, tobramicin, and amikacin) are direct proximal and distal tubular toxins.

Epidem: This is still a relatively frequent cause of toxin-induced AKI in spite of the availability of newer antibiotics. There has been a trend toward using these agents in sicker patients because of emerging drug-resistant pathogens. Preexisting kidney dysfunction and concurrent renal hypoperfusion increase the risk of AKI, as does dosing inappropriately high for renal function. Loop diuretics promote the tubular cell uptake of aminoglycosides and increase the risk.

Pathophys: These drugs are directly toxic to the proximal and distal tubules where they interfere with energy metabolism and make cells more susceptible to ischemic damage.

Sx/Si: Hearing loss, tinnitus, and vestibular dysfunction may be present due to simultaneous ototoxicity.

Crs: The onset of AKI is usually 4–5 days after the initiation of rx. Nonoliguric AKI is usually slow to recover, and some patients will be left with permanent renal impairment.

Cmplc: Ototoxicity can occur at the same time. Irreversible vestibular dysfunction can occur, resulting in a severe lifelong disability even after recovery of renal function. Failure to recover renal function may also occur.

Lab: Serum electrolytes, BUN, Cr, urinalysis. (The classic finding of brown granular casts, also called muddy brown casts, is neither sensitive nor specific.)

Rx: Prevention is critical. Identification of patients at risk for AKI and consideration of alternative antibiotics should be undertaken. Renal hypoperfusion should be corrected if possible. Once daily dosing of aminoglycosides reduces the risk of nephrotoxicity by 25% (Br Med J 1996;312:338).

Amphotericin B-Induced Kidney Injury

(Drug Saf 1990;5:94)

Cause: Amphotericin B is directly toxic to renal tubular cells.

Epidem: Renal toxicity will occur in 30%–80% of the patients treated with this drug. While the frequency of fungal infections has increased, the use of newer antifungal agents has reduced the frequency of this complication. Male gender, concomitant use of cyclosporine, and high amphotericin B dose are risk factors for the development of AKI.

Pathophys: Amphotericin B associates with tubular cell membranes and changes membrane permeability. Interference with macula densa function leads to afferent artery vasoconstriction and sodium wasting (tubuloglomerular feedback). This drug also causes K and Mg wasting. Deoxycholate, an additive used to improve the solubility of amphotericin B, is also directly nephrotoxic. Liposomal amphotericin B is less nephrotoxic.

Si: Azotemia (either oliguric or nonoliguric AKI), hypokalemia, hypomagnesemia, sodium wasting, distal renal tubular acidosis

Crs: Renal recovery occurs slowly after the drug is discontinued. Recovery is frequently incomplete.

Cmplc: During the phase of acute toxicity, complications are related to electrolyte depletion. Long-term incomplete recovery will lead to chronic kidney disease.

Lab: Serum electrolytes including Mg

Rx: Saline loading and maintenance of high urine flow may ameliorate nephrotoxicity. When possible, use of liposomal amphotericin B is preferred.

ACUTE KIDNEY INJURY

Acyclovir Cristaluria and Kidney Injury

(Am J Kidney Dis 2005;45:804)

Cause: Intratubular deposition of acyclovir crystals causes tubular injury.

Epidem: Usually associated with high dose intravenous acyclovir therapy but can occasionally occur with oral acyclovir

Pathophys: Crystals can form in concentrated urine of the patients who are not well hydrated. Acyclovir crystals have been seen in the kidney biopsy specimens in and around renal tubules.

Crs: Toxicity is usually transient and will resolve with discontinuation of acyclovir and hydration.

Lab: Azotemia can develop in the course of acyclovir rx. Acyclovir crystals may be seen in urine.

Rx: Prevention by administration of saline prior to administration of acyclovir

3.8   Myoglobinuric Acute Kidney Injury

(Intensive Care Med 2001;27:803)

Cause: Release of muscle cell contents in traumatic and nontraumatic muscle cell breakdown leads to myoglobinuria, which in turn causes AKI. Causes of rhabdomyolysis are summarized in Table 3.2.

Table 3.2   Causes of Myoglobinuric Acute Kidney Injury

Type of Injury	Causes Associated with This Type of Injury
Traumatic	crush injury, burns
Ischemic	immobility and compression (immobility, coma, anesthesia, drug and alcohol abuse)
Drugs	fibrates and HMG CoA reductase inhibitors (especially when agents from 2 categories are used in combination in patients with impaired drug metabolism)

Table 3.2   Causes of Myoglobinuric Acute Kidney Injury (continued)

Type of Injury	Causes Associated with This Type of Injury
Excessive muscle activity	seizures, extreme exercise (marathon running and others), stimulant abuse (cocaine and amphetamines)
Bacterial infections	clostridia, legionella
Viral infections	coxsackie, adenovirus, influenza
Autoimmune	polymyositis, dermatomyositis
Electrolyte disorders	profound hypokalemia, hypophosphatemia
Genetic	McArdle's disease

Epidem: Trauma and crush injury are important causes from the public health standpoint. In many cases, however, abnormal laboratory studies are seen prior to the recognition of muscle injury. These are often due to ischemia either in the setting of prolonged immobility, severe ischemia due to vascular disease, or drug and alcohol abuse.

Pathophys: Once filtered, heme proteins found in the myoglobin contribute to tubular cell injury via several mechanisms. Heme causes direct proximal tubular toxicity, renal vasoconstriction, and intratubular cast formation.

Sx: Symptoms will be related to the disease that led to muscle injury.

Si: Injured muscles may be tender.

Crs: Depends on the severity of AKI and electrolyte disorders. In particularly severe cases, such as massive crush injuries associated with natural disasters, mortality may be especially high, reaching as high as 15% as was seen in the Marmara earthquake in Turkey in 1999. Hyperkalemia is often a significant contributor to mortality in these cases.

Cmplc: Life-threatening electrolyte disturbances and death due to hyperkalemia. Need for prolonged dialysis or failure to recover renal function may occur.

Lab: Severe and life-threatening hyperkalemia is common, along with hyperphosphatemia and hyperuricemia. Hypocalcemia is seen

ACUTE KIDNEY INJURY

early due to deposition of calcium in injured muscle, while late in the disease, hypercalcemia can be seen as that calcium is released from the injured tissue. Urinary sediment will reveal pigmented granular casts consistent with ATN. Dipstick urinalysis positive for heme combined with the absence of red cells in the sediment suggests myoglobinuria. Urine can be tested directly for the presence of myoglobin.

Rx: Aggressive volume resuscitation is critical for the prevention and management of myoglobinuric AKI. For the victims of disasters who are trapped in the wreckage and have a crushed limb, iv fluid must be started as soon as possible in the field even before they are extricated from the wreckage. Because hyperkalemia is a frequent cause of mortality in these cases, potassium-containing solutions should be avoided. Urine alkalinization can increase the solubility of heme proteins in the renal tubules. Prior to initiation of alkalinization, good urine flow should be established, if possible, by administration of saline. While the use of loop diuretics and mannitol has been advocated in the past, there appears to be little benefit when these agents are added to aggressive saline resuscitation (Ren Fail 1997;19:283). Administration of sodium bicarbonate to anuric and oliguric patients should be avoided as it will lead to metabolic alkalosis, which is not a goal of treatment. Compartment syndrome and severe acute ischemia are surgical emergencies that may require fasciotomy and amputation.

The recently described concept of a renal disaster refers to a period following a natural or a man-made disaster where large numbers of patients with acute kidney injury due to crush injuries and resulting myoglobinuric AKI may require dialysis in a chaotic situation where medical infrastructure may be severely damaged (N Engl J Med 2006;354:1052). Disaster preparation must include plans for transferring victims of crush injuries with AKI to facilities where dialysis is available, as well as managing limited supplies and personnel under difficult circumstances.

3.9   Rapidly Progressive Glomerulonephritis

(J Nephrol 2004;17[suppl 8]:S10)

Introduction: RPGN is an AKI syndrome where aggressive glomerular inflammation and disruption can produce a deterioration of renal function in the course of days to weeks. Glomerular crescent formation is the classic pathologic feature of this disease. The mechanism of crescent formation is shown in Figure 3.1. While

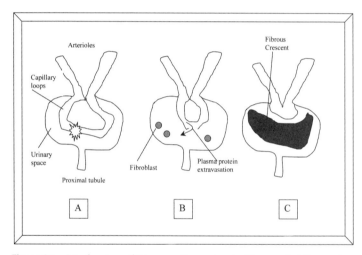

Figure 3.1   Mechanism of Crescent Formation in Crescentic Glomerulonephritis. Initial injury by one of several autoimmune mechanisms leads to the disruption of the glomerular capillary wall and its basement membrane (A). Disruption of the capillary wall allows blood proteins to enter the urinary space, and cellular proliferation may also occur. Cellular proliferation leads to the cellular crescent stage (B). At this point recovery may be possible. If fibroblasts enter a cellular crescent and proliferate, the crescent will progress to become a fibrous crescent (C). When this occurs, recovery of normal glomerular architecture is not possible.

many glomerulonephritis syndromes exist, many do not cause acute inflammation severe enough to disrupt the glomerular architecture and cause the development of crescents and rapid loss of renal function.

Four distinct RPGN syndromes have been recognized and are discussed in this section and in Chapter 4.

1. Antiglomerular Basement Membrane Disease (Goodpasture's Disease)

(J Nephrol 2004;17[suppl 8]:S10)

Cause: Development of autoimmune antibody response to the carboxyl-terminal, noncollagenous domain of type IV collagen. This part of the type IV collagen molecule is sometimes referred to as the Goodpasture antigen.

Epidem: This is a rare disease, which occurs with the frequency of less than 1 per 1 million people per year.

Pathophys: IgG antibodies attach to the glomerular basement membrane and initiate inflammation there. Neutrophils, macrophages, and complement all participate in the subsequent inflammation and glomerular disruption.

In the lung, an additional insult such as tobacco smoking or any other lung problem such as pulmonary edema can expose alveolar basement membrane to circulating antibodies and result in a life-threatening pulmonary hemorrhage.

Sx: Hemoptysis or shortness of breath may occur in the patients with lung involvement. If the disease is renal limited, only the non-specific features of renal failure may be present.

Crs: Untreated disease will rapidly progress to irreversible renal failure. Pulmonary hemorrhage can be rapidly fatal. Pulmonary disease can be somewhat subclinical and occur without overt hemopty-sis. This can present as diffuse lung disease of unclear etiology. Patients who present with a serum Cr of more than 5.7 mg/dL and especially those who require dialysis shortly after presentation have a very poor prognosis for renal recovery even with aggressive treatment, unless concurrent ATN is present.

Cmplc: Death due to massive pulmonary hemorrhage, complications of renal failure such as hyperkalemia and volume overload. Complications of immunosuppressive therapy and plasma exchange treatments can occur.

Lab: Anti-GBM antibody titers will be high. Routine laboratory studies will be consistent with renal failure. Sudden onset of anemia or a precipitous drop in hemoglobin in an already anemic patient should raise the suspicion of pulmonary hemorrhage even in patients without hemoptysis.

ANCA may be positive along with the anti-GBM antibody titers. This disorder is likely to behave more like ANCA vasculitis clinically.

Kidney Bx: Should be performed urgently as soon as safe. Some patients may require dialysis prior to biopsy for the correction of prolonged bleeding time (due to severe uremia) as well as hypertension and volume overload. Immunofluorescence microscopy will reveal the classic finding of ribbon-like IgG glomerular deposits and glomerular crescents.

Xray: CXR and other chest imaging will have diffuse alveolar infiltrates when pulmonary involvement is present.

Rx: Aggressive immunosuppression with pulse iv methylprednisolone (500–1000 mg daily for 3 days followed by daily oral prednisone) can be started in cases with high clinical suspicion even prior to kidney biopsy. Once the diagnosis is established, plasma exchange with human albumin is required to remove the pathogenic antibodies. Cyclophosphamide should be used, along with methylprednisolone, to arrest the production of antibodies. Fresh frozen plasma should be used as replacement fluid during plasma exchange treatments when bleeding is present or around the time of invasive procedures. Appropriate prophylaxis should accompany the immunosuppressive rx, such as *Pneumocystis jirovecii* (formerly *Pneumocystis carinii*) pneumonia prophylaxis, with TMP/SMX and stress ulcer prophylaxis.

Patients who present with a serum Cr of more than 5.7 mg/dL and particularly those who are dialysis dependent from presentation and without pulmonary disease are unlikely to have renal recovery and may not benefit from the very high-risk immunosuppressive treatment. Unfortunately, presentation with advanced renal failure is not uncommon, and a decision not to treat with immunosuppressant therapy, especially in cases where a kidney biopsy reveals severe irreversible damage, may be appropriate.

2. ANCA Vasculitis

(Am J Med 2004;117:39)

Introduction: The name ANCA vasculitis is used to describe a group of disorders with substantial similarities and overlap. While in practice it may often be difficult to differentiate among these conditions, the Chapel Hill Consensus Conference defined 3 distinct disorders: Wegener's granulomatosis, microscopic polyangiitis, and Churg-Strauss syndrome. Distinct clinical features of these disorders are shown in Table 3.3.

Cause: ANCA vasculitides are a group of complex immune mediated disorders with an as yet unclear etiology of immune activation.

Epidem: In the United States, 90% of patients with ANCA vasculitis are white. While the median age of onset is 55, the disease is commonly seen in the very elderly and can occasionally be seen in teenagers.

Pathophys: This is incompletely understood. The cause of the immune activation is unclear. ANCA itself appears to play an active role in the disease, along with a multitude of immune cells.

Table 3.3 Features of Antineutrophil Cytoplasmic Antibody Vasculitides

Manifestation	Wegener's Granulomatosis	Microscopic Polyangiitis	Churg-Strauss Syndrome
Kidney biopsy	Common Global or segmental glomerular crescents and necrosis. Necrotizing arteritis. Granulomatous inflammation	Common Global or segmental glomerular crescents and necrosis	Less common Global or segmental glomerular crescents and necrosis Rare granulomatous inflammation
Immune Deposits	Never	Never	Never
Lungs	Alveolitis Alveolar hemorrhage Granulomas	Alveolitis Alveolar hemorrhage	Asthma Alveolar hemorrhage
Eosinophilia	Occasional	Not present	Always present
Upper airway disease*	Common	Rare	Common
Rash or cutaneous nodules	Sometimes	Sometimes	Sometimes
Peripheral neuropathy	Rare	Sometimes	Common (mononeuritis multiplex)
Myalgias and Arthralgias	Sometimes	Sometimes	Sometimes

*Sinusitis, including granulomatous destruction of bone in Wegener's Granulomatosis, otitis media, permanent hearing loss, ocular inflammation, and subglotic disease.

Sx: Symptoms depend on the site of involvement and the exact nature of the disorder. Wegener's granulomatosis may present with prominent upper respiratory symptoms, while the prominent feature of the Churg-Strauss syndrome is asthma. Presenting

ACUTE KIDNEY INJURY

symptoms are often nonspecific and require consideration of a broad differential diagnosis.

Crs: Untreated ANCA vasculitis has a very poor prognosis. With treatment, a remission is possible for many patients, although relapse is often a threat. Most patients will be left with permanent morbidity, particularly CKD and hearing loss. Five-year survival is approximately 75%. First year mortality is 18%, mostly due to infection.

Cmplc: Treatment-related complications such as infection and drug related toxicity. In particular, neutropenia due to cyclophosphamide is common, and careful monitoring is necessary.

Lab: An elevated ANCA titer in the correct clinical setting is very useful for the diagnosis. ANCA has limited utility in predicting remission and relapse, as it does not correlate perfectly with disease activity; a rise in ANCA titer should be considered to be a risk factor for relapse but not a definite indication that a relapse is occurring. At least 10% of patients with Wegener's granulomatosis are ANCA negative.

Kidney Bx: Biopsy is indicated in many cases. There is controversy as to whether a biopsy is needed in patients with a classic presentation of RPGN and a strongly positive ANCA. The findings will reveal glomerular crescent formation and fibrinoid necrosis. Tubulointerstitial nephritis is common.

Rx: The current standard of care for patients with severe vasculitis that causes RPGN is induction therapy with oral cyclophosphamide at 1.5 mg/kg/d (dose may need to be adjusted for decreased renal function), along with prednisone for 3–6 months, followed by azathioprine 2 mg/kg/d for the maintenance of remission (N Engl J Med 2003;349:3).

Patients receiving oral cyclophosphamide need to be monitored with a complete blood count at least every several wks. Routine prophylaxis with TMP/SMX for *Pneumocystis jirovecii* (formerly *Pneumocystis carinii*) pneumonia is appropriate in most patients. Cyclophosphamide should be stopped in patients who develop neutropenia; it can be resumed at a lower dose after recovery from neutropenia.

Patients with milder respiratory-limited Wegener's granulomatosis or those with Churg-Strauss syndrome may not require treatment with cyclophosphamide. Respiratory-limited Wegener's granulomatosis can be treated with steroids and methotrexate. Milder cases of Churg-Strauss syndrome can be treated with steroids alone.

3. Poststreptococcal Glomerulonephritis

(J Paediatr Child Health 2007;43:446)

Cause: Pharyngitis or skin infection with group A β-hemolytic streptococci.

Epidem: This is a disease of children. In the above reference, which describes an urban population in a developed country, the mean age of children was 8.1 yrs (range 2.6–14.1). This is a much more common condition in rural areas of poor countries.

Pathophys: Streptococcal antigens lead to immune complex formation and glomerular deposition.

Sx/Si: Symptoms typically begin 2–3 wks after the throat or skin infection. Hematuria, described as tea-colored or smoky urine, is a common presenting complaint. Hematuria occurring simultaneously with the sore throat should raise the suspicion of IgA nephropathy. Edema and hypertension are common.

Crs: Most patients will have some degree of renal impairment, but need for dialysis is unusual. Most patients will have a complete renal recovery. Biopsy findings suggestive of severe injury, such as crescents, often heal completely and do not lead to bad outcomes.

ACUTE KIDNEY INJURY

Cmplc: Renal failure requiring dialysis, severe hypertension with end-organ damage (eg, seizures). After recovery, persistent hematuria lasting from several months to several years can be seen in some patients.

Lab: In addition to glomerular hematuria and proteinuria, low C3 with normal C4 is usually seen. Elevated titer of antibodies against streptolysin O (ASO) is usually present. The infection itself is likely to be resolved, and cultures are likely to be negative.

Kidney Bx: Light microscopy will reveal acute proliferative glomerulonephritis. Crescents can be seen along with many neutrophils. Immunofluorescence microscopy reveals deposits of IgG and C3. Electron microscopy will reveal subendothelial deposits as well as the large subepithelial humps, which are a classic finding in this condition.

Rx: Antibiotic treatment of streptococcal infections does not prevent poststreptococcal glomerulonephritis, but it may lessen its severity. Patients who present with glomerulonephritis should be treated with antibiotics, if not already done. Supportive treatment for edema and hypertension is often required. Immunosuppressive treatment is not necessary, as recovery of renal function will usually occur over several weeks.

4. Crescentic IgA Nephropathy

Crescentic IgA nephropathy is discussed in Chapter 4.8.

3.10   Acute Interstitial Nephritis

(Am Fam Physician 2003;67:2527)

Cause: Immunologic hypersensitivity reaction. The precipitating factor is often a drug or an infectious agent. For a complete list of causes see Table 3.4.

Table 3.4   Common Causes of Acute Interstitial Nephritis

Drugs
  Antibiotics
      Penicillins
      Cephalosporins
      Ciprofloxacin
      Sulfonamides
      Rifampin
      other Antibiotics
  NSAIDs
      Aspirin
      Ibuprofen
      Naproxen
      Most other NSAIDs
      Mesalamine
      Sulfasalazine
  Other Drugs
      Allopurinol
      Azathioprine
      Omeprazole
      others
Typical Bacteria
  Escherichia coli
  Brucella
  Campylobacter
  Staphylococcus
  Streptococcus
  others
Atypical Bacteria
  Mycobacterium tuberculoses
  Legionella
  Mycoplasma
  Chlamydia
Viruses
  Cytomegalovirus
  Hantavirus
  Herpes Viruses

ACUTE KIDNEY INJURY

Table 3.4   Common Causes of Acute Interstitial Nephritis (continued)

HIV
Hepatitis B
others
Autoimmune Diseases
  Sarcoidosis
  Sjögren's syndrome
  Systemic Lupus Erythematosus
  ANCA Vasculitis
Renal Transplant Associated
  Cellular Rejection
  BK Polyoma Virus
Malignant Cell Infiltration
  Leukemia
  Lymphoma
  Idiopathic

Epidem: This is a rare cause of AKI, unless AKI related to a newly prescribed drug is being investigated.

Pathophys: The precipitating antigen that is often extrarenal (drug or infection related) leads to inflammation in the interstitial compartment of the kidney by a variety of incompletely understood immune mechanisms.

In some cases of NSAID-induced AIN, patients can present with a simultaneous nephrotic syndrome with a minimal change glomerular lesion.

Sx: Often nonspecific, fever, rash and arthralgias may be present.

Si: Rash

Crs: Drug-induced AIN is usually associated with complete renal recovery, although it may take months. Outcome of AIN in infectious and other systemic conditions will depend on the outcome of the underlying condition.

Cmplc: Electrolyte disorders, volume overload, or symptomatic uremia. Recovery of renal function may be incomplete with residual CKD.

Lab: The definitive diagnosis is only possible with a kidney biopsy. Pyuria and wbc casts can be present. The utility of urine eosinophils for diagnosis of AIN is limited, as they can be present in a number of conditions.

Rx: Removal of the inciting agent or treatment of the underlying disease is the cornerstone of treatment of AIN. In drug-induced AIN, a brief course of prednisone at 1 mg/kg may hasten the recovery of renal function, but it does not change the eventual outcome. Steroids appear to be even less effective in the treatment of NSAID-induced AIN.

3.11 Acute Kidney Injury in Decompensated Congestive Heart Failure

(Am J Nephrol 2007;27:55)

Cause: Reduction in renal blood flow due to poor cardiac output with resultant activation of counterproductive neurohormonal mechanisms.

Many patients in this clinical setting have pre-existing CKD and suffer AKI superimposed on CKD.

Epidem: Depending on the definition of AKI, it may complicate 16%–53% of hospital admissions for decompensated CHF. When AKI is defined as an increase in serum Cr of 0.5 mg/dL, the incidence of AKI is about 20%.

Predictors for the development of AKI associated with CHF decompensation are:

- Higher baseline serum creatinine
- Hyponatremia (admission sodium of less than 136 mEq/L increases the risk of AKI by a factor of 12)

- Diastolic dysfunction
- Admission serum creatinine of greater than 3 mg/dL

The data regarding the risk of AKI in patients who received ACEIs and ARBs prior to admission are conflicting. In some studies, the risk of AKI in patients randomized to the ACEI groups was quite high and was associated with increased mortality (Am Heart J 1999;138:849). There are conflicting data regarding the effect of previous diuretic therapy on the risk of AKI during the hospitalization. The degree of LV dysfunction has little effect on the risk of AKI during hospitalization for decompensated CHF.

Pathophys: Reduced renal blood flow superimposed on pre-existing chronic renal dysfunction.

Sx: Breathlessness and edema due to heart failure.

Si: Edema, rales, and jugular venous distension.

Crs/Cmplc: Most cases of AKI in patients hospitalized for decompensated CHF occur around hospital day 4. Development of AKI at least doubles the risk of death during that admission from about 4% during a heart failure admission without AKI to about 9% in patients who do develop AKI. In one study, the risk of death in decompensated heart failure patients with AKI was 7.5 times higher than in those who did not suffer AKI (JAMA 2005;293:572). Development of AKI during an admission for CHF prolongs the length of stay by about 3 days.

Lab: Given the high risk of AKI in patients admitted for decompensated CHF, renal function should be monitored frequently.

Rx: The usual care in this setting involves intravenous diuretics several times a day or by continuous infusion. Thiazide diuretics are often used in combination with loop diuretics. Prevention and treatment of AKI during admissions for decompensated CHF should center on avoiding inadvertent hypovolemia from excessive diuretic administration. While ACEIs and ARBs are typically discontinued in this setting, the evidence that they slow down the recovery of renal function once AKI occurs is controversial.

Nesiritide is the natriuretic peptide indicated for the rx of decompensated heart failure. Nesiritide is not indicated for the treatment of AKI in CHF patients until more information is available regarding the renal effects of this drug.

Ultrafiltration for patients who could have been treated with diuretics has been a subject of substantial recent interest, and specialized equipment aimed at delivering ultrafiltration therapy for patients with decompensated CHF is available. Ultrafiltration does not activate as many counterproductive neurohormonal mechanisms and delivers more predictable fluid removal. The UNLOAD trial demonstrated a significant reduction in rehospitalization rates in patients treated with ultrafiltration as compared to diuretics. This study was conducted in patients whose renal failure was not so severe as to require dialysis. Ultrafiltration and diuretics produced similar amounts of renal dysfunction. This may be a promising new treatment for decompensated CHF. It is important to emphasize that these new therapies are directed at patients who can be successfully treated with diuretics. Patients with severe renal impairment and indications for dialysis should be treated with dialysis (J Am Coll Cardiol 2007;49:675).

3.12 Abdominal Compartment Syndrome

(Curr Opin Crit Care 2005;11:333)

Cause: Reduced renal perfusion probably due to venous compression stemming from increased intra-abdominal pressure in the setting of trauma, massive volume resuscitation, tense abdominal surgical closure, pancreatitis, peritonitis, massive ascites, or bowel obstruction.

Epidem: Most often seen in trauma or abdominal surgery patients.

Pathophys: Elevated intra-abdominal pressure leads to compression of visceral organs, respiratory and cardiac compromise, as well as intestinal, hepatic, and renal ischemia. The mechanism of renal ischemia in this syndrome is incompletely understood, but it is likely related to vascular (probably venous) compression.

Si: Tensely distended abdomen and low urine output

Crs: Oliguric AKI will persist for as long as intra-abdominal pressure remains elevated.

Lab: Azotemia and electrolyte disturbances consistent with AKI

Special Test: Measurement of intra-abdominal pressure can be easily accomplished by placing 50 ml of saline into the urinary bladder and clamping the drainage tube of a regular Foley catheter. Following the instillation of saline, the sampling port of the Foley catheter can be connected to a pressure transducer used for the measurement of CVP, which is readily available at the bedside of any critically ill patient. The transducer should be zeroed at the level of the bladder (Crit Care Med 1987;15:1140).

Usually abdominal compartment syndrome is not present when the intra-abdominal pressure is less than 10 mm Hg. The adverse sequelae of this condition can begin occurring when the intra-abdominal pressure begins to exceed 12 mm Hg. Clinically significant abdominal compartment syndrome is always present when intra-abdominal pressure exceeds 25 mm Hg.

Rx: Surgical decompression is often required. In selected cases, decompression can be accomplished via paracentesis.

3.13 Acute Kidney Injury Due to Cholesterol Embolization

(Kidney Int 2006;69:1308)

Cause: Embolization of cholesterol crystals from the aorta and renal arteries into small renal vessels. This can be due to endovascular procedures, particularly cardiac catheterization or renal artery procedures; vascular surgery; or anticoagulation. Spontaneous cholesterol embolism has also been described. There is also a subset of patients in whom periodic spontaneous embolization leads to CKD.

Epidem: This is a disease of older individuals undergoing the above described procedures or anticoagulation.

Pathophys: Initially, crystals obstructing small arteries cause transient thrombosis with subsequent inflammation and permanent vascular obstruction.

Sx: In addition to sx related to renal failure, patients may experience symptoms due to embolization to other organ and body areas, such as lower extremity pain and abdominal pain due to intestinal ischemia.

Si: Diminished peripheral pulses, livedo reticularis, or rash that may even resemble vasculitic rash may be seen in some individuals.

Crs: Depends on the severity of the event. Most patients will be left with some degree of permanent renal impairment. Some individuals may experience very slow renal recovery even after requiring dialysis, while others will relentlessly progress to end-stage renal disease.

Cmplc: Severe hypertension, complications of embolization to other locations such as intestine or toes.

Lab: Time course of the onset of renal failure after endovascular procedures is critical. Contrast-associated nephropathy usually occurs shortly after the procedure. Contrast-induced AKI usually has a spontaneous recovery. Cholesterol embolization syndrome causes subacute kidney injury over a number of weeks. Oliguria and rapid onset of renal failure is seen in only the most severe cases, where embolization to other organs and extremities is easily apparent.

ACUTE KIDNEY INJURY

Kidney Bx: In most cases, the diagnosis can be made by history and by observing the involvement of other organs. Kidney biopsy should be necessary in only 20% of cases.

Rx: Further endovascular procedures should be avoided. If cholesterol embolization was precipitated by anticoagulation, anticoagulation should be stopped and further anticoagulation avoided. There may be a role for HMG-CoA reductase inhibitor (statin) therapy following a cholesterol embolization event.

3.14 Hepatorenal Syndrome

(Clin Liver Dis 2006;10:371)

Cause: Hemodynamic alterations that accompany severe liver disease with portal hypertension lead to renal failure in the absence of parenchymal kidney disease. While HRS may occur spontaneously, it is often precipitated by an infection, such as sepsis or spontaneous bacterial peritonitis, or by a large volume paracentesis. Very edematous patients with significant ascites and hypervolemic hyponatremia are at especially high risk of developing HRS.

Classification: HRS is classified into type 1 and type 2. Type 1 HRS patients have a rapid rise in serum creatinine to over 2.5 mg/dL in less than 2 wks. Type 2 HRS is a less severe form with rises of creatinine to at least 1.5 mg/dL that may occur over a longer period of time.

Epidem: The disease occurs almost exclusively in patients with advanced cirrhosis, although it can occasionally be seen in patients with alcoholic hepatitis or acute liver disease due to any cause.

Pathophys: Intense renal arterial vasoconstriction in combination with decreased cardiac output and splanchnic vasodilatation lead to a dramatic reduction in renal perfusion.

Si: Signs of liver failure and portal hypertension, particularly massive ascites.

Crs: Survival is usually poor. In type 1 HRS, median survival is measured in weeks, and most patients die within 2–3 months from the onset of renal failure. Patients with type 2 HRS have a median survival of 6 months.

Cmplc: Patients requiring dialysis will be at risk of numerous complications, particularly hypotension and multiple hospitalizations for a variety of complications (Ren Fail 2004;26:563).

Lab: Low urine sodium in a patient who has undergone withdrawal of diuretics and has been adequately volume expanded, preferably with albumin, is consistent with HRS.

Xray: It may be reasonable to rule out obstruction of the urinary tract with renal ultrasound since it can also cause low urine sodium.

Rx: Given the high mortality rate of HRS, patients suspected of having this condition should undergo intensive medical management from the time HRS is suspected, which should include:

- Admission to a ward where careful monitoring is possible.
- Discontinuation of all diuretics.
- Other causes of AKI, such as sepsis and urinary tract obstruction, should be ruled out with a careful H&P and renal ultrasound.
- Diagnostic paracentesis to rule out SBP, which is a common cause of HRS.
- Volume expansion, including administration of 40 g of albumin.
- The monitoring of the volume status with CVP measurement should be considered.
- Referral to a liver transplantation program.
- One of the recognized vasoconstriction protocols should be considered after volume expansion has been accomplished:

- Midodrine at 5–7.5 mg po tid and octreotide 100–200 ug subcutaneously tid have been shown to be beneficial in a small study (Hepatology 1999;29:1690).
- IV terlipressin, which is not available in the United States, with a starting dose of 1 mg/d, which may be titrated to 12 mg/d, has been demonstrated in a small randomized trial to be superior to placebo in improving renal function (J Gastroenterol Hepatol 2003;18:152).
- TIPS has been evaluated in a small trial in combination with midodrine and octreotide and was found to be beneficial in allowing a better recovery of renal function than medical therapy alone (Hepatology 2004;40:55).
- Dialysis is likely to lead to multiple severe complications and poor survival in this setting. Careful consideration of risks and benefits will be necessary prior to initiation of dialysis in HRS patients (Ren Fail 2004;26:563).

3.15 Multiple Myeloma-Associated Acute Kidney Injury

(Arch Intern Med 1998;158:1889)

Introduction: MM can be associated with a variety of renal lesions that can cause both AKI and chronic glomerular and interstitial lesions. The issues related to a number of glomerular lesions that can be caused by plasma cell disorders are presented in sections 4.11, 4.12, and 4.13. This section will describe AKI that can occur due to or in association with multiple myeloma.

Cause: While many patients diagnosed with MM will develop renal dysfunction, only a minority will have the classic lesion of cast nephropathy, also called myeloma kidney. Many patients with MM will develop AKI due to volume depletion, sepsis, or hypercalcemia-induced ATN, or NSAID and other drug-induced renal injury.

Epidem: MM is a disease of older individuals. Many patients present with some degree of reversible renal dysfunction at the time of diagnosis of MM. Approximately 25% of patients presenting with MM will have renal dysfunction. In 10% of cases, AKI is severe enough to require dialysis at presentation, and many of these patients do not recover enough renal function to survive without dialysis.

Pathophys: In patients with cast nephropathy, freely filtered light chains, which are prone to cast formation, will combine with Tamm-Horsfall protein in the distal tubules and form casts there.

Hypercalcemia causes AKI via several mechanisms, which include the following: intrarenal vasoconstriction, volume depletion due to a sodium and water wasting distal defect, and tubular obstruction by crystals and rapidly developing nephrocalcinosis (see Chapter 1.6).

Sx: Symptoms are usually nonspecific. Back pain is frequent in patients with multiple myeloma.

Crs: The outcome of MM-associated AKI is variable. AKI due to dehydration, sepsis, or hypercalcemia has a good prognosis. The chance of recovery in patients who present with cast nephropathy (myeloma kidney) and requirement for dialysis is poor. In one series, only 15% of the patients who needed dialysis at presentation had recovery with treatment.

Cmplc: Related to dialysis and chemotherapy

Lab: Findings of hypercalcemia, anemia, and renal failure should raise the suspicion of MM. Low AG can be present due to the cationic nature of the paraprotein. Bone marrow biopsy is required to diagnose MM.

In cases of MM with filtered light chains, dipstick UA may be negative even when massive amounts of light chains are filtered and present in urine. The absence of dipstick proteinuria does not rule out myeloma kidney, and testing for urinary protein should be performed with sulfosalicylic acid.

Xray: Skeletal survey may reveal lytic bone lesions.

Rx: Many patients will have hypovolemia, which should be corrected with saline. Hypercalcemia should be treated with volume expansion and forced diuresis with furosemide (see Chapter 1.6). Use of bisphosphonates, such as zoledronic acid, should be considered in hypercalcemic patients at a dose appropriate for the degree of renal dysfunction. Caution is required as all bisphosphonates have been demonstrated to cause ATN, particularly when administered in high doses. High dose pamidronate can cause nephrotic syndrome due to collapsing FSGS.

The role of plasma exchange is controversial. While a randomized trial demonstrated no benefit, it did not base treatment on histological diagnosis of cast nephropathy (Ann Intern Med 2005;143:777). It is possible that some patients with cast nephropathy could benefit from chemotherapy combined with plasma exchange treatments.

3.16   Acute Kidney Injury Due to Tumor Lysis Syndrome (Uric Acid Nephropathy)

(Am J Med 2004;116:546)

Cause: Hematological malignancy. The syndrome often occurs in patients with a large tumor burden. Most cases occur after chemotherapy or radiation. Some cases are spontaneous.

Epidem: The frequency of this complication is unknown.

Pathophys: Tumor cell lysis leads to the release of large amounts of potassium, phosphate, and uric acid into plasma. The rate of release of these substances may exceed the ability to excrete them, especially in patients with pre-existing CKD. Many patients with serious malignant disorders may be unwell and volume depleted for a variety of reasons. These patients have low urine flow rates, and uric acid crystals may precipitate in their renal tubules leading to tubular obstruction and acute renal failure. Hyperphosphatemia may lead to hypocalcemia and tissue and renal calcium deposition. Hyperkalemia always develops first, followed by the hyperphosphatemia. Hyperuricemia typically develops last, as there is a delay between the release of DNA from the lysed cells and its conversion to uric acid.

Sx/Si: Related to malignancy and renal failure. Hypocalcemia may cause muscle cramps, tetany, cardiac arrhythmia, and seizures.

Crs: The course of this condition depends on the severity of electrolyte disturbances and AKI.

Cmplc: Arrhythmias due to hyperkalemia and hypocalcemia and AKI.

Lab: Hyperkalemia, hyperuricemia, and hyperphosphatemia, along with variable degrees of hypocalcemia, will be seen.

When AKI develops, a spot urine uric acid to creatinine ratio can help make the diagnosis of uric acid nephropathy. When the spot urine uric acid to creatinine ratio is greater than 1, it is consistent with uric acid nephropathy. Spot urine uric acid ratios less than 0.75 suggest another cause of renal failure.

Rx: Several interventions can be effective in the management of this disorder.

- Volume expansion with isotonic saline will help prevent AKI due to tumor lysis syndrome by maintaining good urine flow, which will facilitate excretion of potassium and uric acid. Volume expansion should be initiated prior to chemotherapy for patients at risk of this condition.
- Hyperkalemia is managed with administration of calcium to stabilize myocardial membranes. This is particularly important, as hypocalcemia can be present due to renal failure and hyperphosphatemia. Insulin and dextrose can help with short-term management of hyperkalemia and sodium polystyrene

(kayexalate), or RRT may be needed long-term (see Chapter 1.4).

- Hyperphosphatemia can be managed with RRT and phosphate binders.
- Hypocalcemia correction may not be needed in asymptomatic patients without hyperkalemia. If symptoms are present, calcium should be administered with caution to avoid tissue precipitation of calcium phosphate.
- Treatment of hyperuricemia should include therapies that prevent formation of uric acid along with therapies that increase its excretion.
  - Urine alkalinization increases solubility of uric acid. This will only be effective if adequate urine flow can be accomplished with volume resuscitation first. Urine pH > 7 is the goal. Caution should be taken to avoid induction of metabolic alkalosis in patients who are unable to excrete adequate volumes of alkaline urine due to renal impairment. Metabolic alkalosis will increase the chances of tissue precipitation of calcium phosphate.
  - Allopurinol reduces uric acid levels in patients with tumor lysis syndrome, but it takes several days to lower the uric acid levels.
  - Rasburicase (recombinant urate oxidase) rapidly catalyzes the conversion of uric acid to the much more soluble allantoin. Rasburicase will allow the control of uric acid levels within several hours instead of several days with allopurinol.
- If RRT is needed, intermittent hemodialysis will allow for rapid correction of hyperkalemia and hyperuricemia. Control of phosphorous is more difficult and may take several dialysis treatments.

3.17   Thrombotic Microangiopathies

Introduction: The term *thrombotic microangiopathy* (TMA) is used to describe several disorders with a common pathogenesis. TTP and HUS share a common feature, which is the presence of microangiopathic hemolytic anemia. Microangiopathic hemolytic anemia involves formation of intraluminal thrombi that consume platelets. The thrombi then lead to destruction of red blood cells, which leads to a hemolytic anemia with the characteristic finding of schistocytes on the peripheral smear. While there are significant similarities between these disorders, they are discussed separately below, in accordance with the traditional classification.

Thrombotic Thrombocytopenic Purpura

(Hematol Oncol Clin North Am 2007;21:609)

Cause: TTP in previously healthy individuals is usually caused by the development of autoantibodies against the metalloprotease ADAMTS13, which regulates the activity of VWF in the coagulation cascades. Therefore, the condition previously referred to as idiopathic TTP is actually an autoimmune condition caused by autoimmunity to ADAMTS13.

There are several other conditions that can lead to the common pathway of endothelial injury that is similar to the endothelial injury caused by the ADAMTS13 deficiency and result in a similar presentation. These include HIV disease, SLE, and possibly, pregnancy. The issue of the association of TTP with pregnancy is controversial, as TTP is more common in young women and therefore may occasionally present around the time of pregnancy. There is an inherited form of TTP as well.

A drug-induced form of this disorder is seen with ticlopidine, cyclosporine, and tacrolimus. Cyclosporine- and tacrolimus-associated TMA in kidney transplant recipients may have different features, as the disease is often limited to the renal allograft.

ACUTE KIDNEY INJURY

Cancer-associated TTP has been described especially in cases of advanced metastatic disease. The pathogenesis is likely related to endothelial damage by tumor cells. Almost any cancer can be associated with TTP.

Cancer treatment with mitomycin causes TMA in 2%–10% of patients who receive this drug, particularly at high doses. Other chemotherapeutic agents have been associated with TMA as well. They most likely cause direct endothelial injury.

Epidem: The epidemiology of TTP is greatly affected by the baseline prevalence of HIV in the community. In HIV prevalent areas, 50% of TTP cases may be HIV related. In general, TTP is more common in young and middle-aged women. TTP is more common among blacks. The female-to-male predominance may be as high as 3:1.

Pathophys: Different disorders in this group have different initial mechanisms.

In autoimmune (idiopathic) TTP, deficiency of the metallo-protease ADAMTS13 leads to impaired degradation of the VWF multimers. Subsequently, large VWF multimers combine with platelets to form thrombi. This leads to microvascular thrombosis and ischemia of the involved organs along with mechanical hemolysis of the red cells and schistocyte formation.

Ticlopidine causes ADAMTS13 deficiency, while cyclosporine and tacrolimus probably cause direct endothelial injury.

Sx/Si: While the classic pentad of thrombocytopenia, fever, mental status changes, renal dysfunction, and hemolytic anemia is frequently discussed in this setting, all 5 findings are actually rarely present. For example, only 50% of the patients will have fever on presentation. Neurological symptoms are varied in severity and can range from a headache to coma.

Crs: Untreated TTP is usually fatal within days. If the diagnosis is made in time and plasma exchange treatment is initiated, most patients will survive the acute illness, but some will suffer a relapse.

Cmplc: Related to plasma exchange and immunosuppressive treatment. Anaphylaxis to FFP is the single most feared complication of plasma exchange. Failure to recover renal function is uncommon, but it has been observed.

Lab: Anemia, thrombocytopenia, and schistocytes on the peripheral smear are the classic findings. Undetectable haptoglobin is more sensitive for the presence of hemolysis than is elevated LDH. Indirect hyperbilirubinemia and elevated reticulocyte count will also be seen. Lab findings consistent with renal failure will be present along with possible hematuria and proteinuria.

Rx: Plasma exchange with FFP is the mainstay of therapy in this disease. Plasma replaces the missing ADAMTS13 enzyme. Exchange with cryoprecipitate poor FFP has the theoretical advantage of having fewer VWF multimers; however, an early underpowered study did not demonstrate an advantage to cryoprecipitate poor FFP (Br J Haematol 2005;129:79). Plasma infusion should be considered when plasma exchange is not immediately available. Relapses are treated with plasma exchange.

The role of immunosuppressive therapy with any agent for this autoimmune disease has not been defined, although multiple agents have been tried, particularly in refractory cases.

Women with a history of TTP who are considering pregnancy should be counseled that the disease might recur during pregnancy.

TMA due to cyclosporine, tacrolimus, or other drugs that are likely to cause direct endothelial injury is best treated with withdrawal of the offending agent.

Hemolytic Uremic Syndrome

(Am Fam Physician 2006;74:991)

Cause: Diarrhea positive HUS is caused by infection with shiga toxin-producing *Escherichia coli*. There is also a diarrhea negative (atypical) HUS, which has been associated with *Streptococcus pneumoniae* and other infections.

Epidem: This is a disease of children under 10 years old. There are sporadic cases and outbreaks related to contaminated food, particularly undercooked ground beef contaminated with *E. coli* 0157:H7.

Pathophys: After ingestion, enterohemorrhagic *E. coli* bind to intestinal cells and cause their death, leading to bloody diarrhea and allowing the toxin to enter the circulation where it causes damage to the endothelial and other cells in the target organs.

Sx: Diarrhea

Crs: Spontaneous recovery is common with supportive treatment.

Cmplc: Failure to recover renal function, residual CKD

Lab: Anemia, thrombocytopenia, and evidence of hemolysis. Stool culture will be positive for shiga toxin-producing *E. coli* 0157:H7. Labs will be consistent with renal failure; elevated wbc count.

Rx: Usually only supportive treatment is needed. RRT may be needed if indications develop. Antibiotics may be harmful.

3.18   Acute Kidney Injury During Pregnancy

(Crit Care Med 2005;33:S372)

Cause: AKI occurring during each stage of pregnancy has its own differential diagnosis:

- Earlier pregnancy
  - Volume depletion due to hyperemesis gravidarum

- ATN due to septic abortion (usually due to illegal abortion but may occur after therapeutic abortion)
- Later pregnancy
  - Pre-eclampsia, eclampsia, HELLP syndrome
  - Acute fatty liver of pregnancy
  - TTP
  - Hemorrhage
  - Pyelonephritis
  - Urinary tract obstruction
    - Stones
    - Gravid uterus with multiple gestations
    - Maternal urinary tract abnormalities may predispose to obstruction

Epidem: This is now a fairly rare condition, which complicates less than 5% of all pregnancies.

Pathophys: Varies widely by cause. It is generally believed that the normal renal physiology of pregnancy predisposes pregnant women to AKI. In pregnancy, all of the mechanisms that can lead to increased renal blood flow are maximally activated, and therefore, there is no further compensatory response available to increase renal blood flow if needed.

Crs: Depends on the cause. General improvements in prenatal care have reduced the incidence of this complication, but once it occurs the mortality has been reported to be as high as 30% in some studies. Complete renal recovery is common.

Xray: Substantial dilatation of the renal collecting systems is normal in pregnancy, particularly on the right side, which leads to difficulties with the potential diagnosis of obstruction. When the suspicion of obstructive AKI is strong and other causes are unlikely, percutaneous nephrostomy followed by observation of renal function may be the only option. This is rarely necessary.

ACUTE KIDNEY INJURY

Rx: Treatment is disease specific. Should RRT be indicated, anecdotal evidence points to a benefit from earlier initiation of dialysis and higher doses of RRT.

3.19 Acute Kidney Injury Due to Obstruction of the Urinary Tract

Cause: Obstructive AKI occurs when the urethra or both ureters are obstructed. In individuals with 2 normal kidneys, obstruction of a single ureter will not lead to AKI.

Obstruction of a renal transplant or a solitary kidney is an emergency, as the AKI will occur promptly, particularly in cases of complete obstruction. The causes of urinary tract obstruction are listed in Table 3.5.

Table 3.5   Common Causes of Urinary Tract Obstruction

Obstruction of the Ureters

Intrinsic to Urinary System
  Stones
  Papillary necrosis
  Blood clots
  Tumors
      Renal cell tumors
      Transitional cell tumors
      Benign tumors
  Functional
      Vesico-ureteric reflux
  Congenital
      Ureteropelvic junction obstruction
  Structures
      After instrumentation
      Schistosomiasis
  Unique to kidney transplant
      Stenosis of the ureteroneocystostomy

Table 3.5   Common Causes of Urinary Tract Obstruction (continued)

Extrinsic
  Pregnancy*
  Tumors
      Cervical cancer
      Prostate cancer
      Lymphoma
  Idiopathic
      Retroperitoneal fibrosis
  Vascular
      Abdominal aortic aneurism
      Aberrant arteries
  Retroperitoneal hematoma
  Radiation therapy
  Unique to kidney transplant
      Compression by lymphocele

Obstruction of the urethra

Prostate
  Benign prostatic hypertrophy
  Prostate cancer
Bladder
      Stones
      Clots
      Schistosomiasis

  Neurogenic Bladder
      Diabetes
      Spinal cord injury
      Multiple sclerosis
      Anticholinergic drugs
Urethra
  Stones
  Stricture
  Blood clots
  Phimosis
  Meatal stenosis

*Right ureter is classically more involved than the left one.

Epidem: Most cases of bilateral ureter obstruction are caused by cancer. Obstruction of the urethra by an enlarged prostate is a common cause of obstruction in older men.

Pathophys: Obstruction leads to elevation of renal tubular pressure and eventual decline in GFR. Following the relief of obstruction, numerous defects in renal concentrating ability and electrolyte handling occur.

Si: There is wide variability in the presenting symptoms of urinary tract obstruction. While distension of the bladder and the ureters commonly cause pain, some patients will be asymptomatic. Acute obstruction of a ureter causes the classic renal colic with severe flank pain radiating to the groin, labia, or testes.

Crs: If obstruction is relieved early (several days), prompt renal recovery will occur; prolonged obstruction will lead to incomplete recovery and may result in CKD.

Cmplc: Urinary tract obstruction predisposes to the development of urinary tract infections. Hematuria may be present when obstruction is caused by a tumor. Relief of obstruction can result in uncontrolled postobstructive diuresis, which can lead to volume depletion and electrolyte disturbances.

Lab: Urinalysis will have widely varied findings depending on the cause of obstruction and associated conditions.

Xray: Ultrasound is the first line test for the diagnosis of obstruction. The finding of hydronephrosis suggests obstruction of the urinary tract anywhere below the kidney. Often the cause of obstruction cannot be visualized by ultrasound. CT can be used to demonstrate kidney stones, tumors, lymphadenopathy, and retroperitoneal fibrosis.

In some cases, hydronephrosis may not develop even though the kidney is obstructed. This is seen early in the course of the obstruction or when the kidney is encased in tumor. Nuclear diuretic renogram (MAG3 scan with furosemide) can be used to diagnose obstruction in the setting where a false negative ultrasound is suspected but some renal function is present. The nuclear pharmaceutical will be taken up by the kidneys and then rapidly excreted into the urine. Failure to do so suggests obstruction of the urinary tract.

Pregnant patients have dilatation of the urinary collecting systems as a normal response to pregnancy. Caution is required in this situation as the appearance of the dilated collecting system on renal ultrasound may be difficult to interpret as normal or abnormal in a pregnant patient.

Rx: Obstruction of the bladder is relieved with a Foley catheter or a suprapubic tube if the urethral catheter cannot be placed. Ureteral stents or percutaneous nephrostomy tubes can be used to relieve obstruction of the ureters. Nephrostomy tubes are easier to use emergently as they require only local anesthesia, and there is a greater likelihood of success, as certain malignant conditions can make placement of a ureteral stent impossible.

Once obstruction is relieved and renal recovery begins to occur, the definitive treatment can be undertaken if possible. Large urine output after relief of the obstruction can be due to excretion of accumulated fluid and solutes. Inappropriate postobstructive diuresis due to failure of urine concentration and other forms of tubular dysfunction can occur as well. Therapy of the latter condition involves careful monitoring of the urine output and electrolytes and replacement of urine output with 0.45% saline and electrolytes as appropriate.

Chapter 4
Glomerular Diseases

4.1 Approach to a Patient with Glomerular Disease

(Aust Fam Physician 2005;34:907)

Glomerular disorders can present in a variety of clinical settings with varying degrees of severity. Recognition of the pattern of disease is the critical first step in approaching the diagnosis and management of glomerular conditions. The following features may be present in varying combinations:

- Glomerular hematuria
- Proteinuria
- Edema
- Impaired GFR
- Hypertension

Once the presence of glomerular disease has been recognized, the following general considerations apply:

- Hematuria may be due to kidney or urological disease while proteinuria is usually due to a disturbance within the kidneys.
- Dysmorphic red blood cells and red cells casts indicate glomerular hematuria.
- Older individuals and those with a tobacco smoking history are at risk of urological malignancy and should not be automatically assumed to have glomerular hematuria, as this may lead to the delay of diagnosis of malignant urological disease.
- Glomerular disorders that are likely to produce renal impairment in the near future will typically include hematuria, proteinuria, and hypertension.

- AKI occurring in association with new onset glomerular disease is consistent with RPGN. This is a medical emergency, which usually requires hospitalization to ensure an efficient diagnostic workup and prompt initiation of treatment. (RPGN is discussed in detail in Chapter 3.3.)
- New onset of proteinuria (either nephrotic or subnephrotic) can usually be safely investigated in the outpatient setting.
- The reagent used in dipstick urinalysis will only detect albuminuria. Bence-Jones proteinuria due to MM can be missed by dipstick urinalysis.
- Spot urine protein to creatinine ratio allows for the rapid determination of the severity of proteinuria in individuals of average muscle mass without the need for cumbersome 24-hr urine collections. The protein to creatinine ratio is also an excellent way to monitor the response to treatment in proteinuric illnesses. Since an average size individual produces about 1 g of creatinine per day, spot urine protein concentration measured in mg/dL divided by spot urine creatinine concentration measured in mg/dL will approximately equal spot urine protein excretion in grams per day.
- Diabetes is the most common cause of proteinuria and nephrotic range proteinuria in the developed world.
- Patients with diabetic retinopathy and proteinuria are very likely to have diabetic kidney disease and generally do not require a biopsy for diagnostic certainty (see Chapter 4.3).
- Kidney biopsy is often required for correct diagnosis and treatment of non-diabetic glomerular diseases.
- The procedure is performed with a 15- or 16-gauge automatic biopsy device with ultrasound guidance and local anesthesia. Sedation is generally not necessary.
- Planning for a kidney biopsy includes the following steps:
  - Informed consent
  - Discontinuation of aspirin and other antiplatelet agents and anticoagulants.

- Renal ultrasound to verify the presence of 2 kidneys without gross defects that would make the biopsy unsafe (multiple cysts, tumors, abscesses)
- Coagulation workup (PT, PTT, platelet count, bleeding time if severe uremia present)
- Abnormal PT and PTT must be worked up prior to proceeding; platelet count must be greater than 100,000 per mm^3.
- Prolonged bleeding time due to uremia can be partially corrected by administration of desmopressin 0.3 mcg/kg prior to the biopsy.
- Indications for kidney biopsy include:
  - Nephrotic syndrome in adults (except clear cases of diabetic nephropathy)
  - Significant non-nephrotic proteinuria
  - Hematuria and proteinuria
  - RPGN
  - Unexplained AKI
- Contraindications for kidney biopsy
  - Uncontrolled bleeding diathesis
  - Active infection (pyelonephritis)
  - Uncontrolled hypertension
  - Uremia (prolonged bleeding time)
  - Renal tumor
  - Multiple cysts
  - Solitary kidney (except kidney transplant)
  - Severe obesity
- While most complications occur during the first 8 hrs following a kidney biopsy, an overnight bed rest is generally recommended.
- The principal complication of an ultrasound guided biopsy is bleeding, and the following general considerations apply:
  - It is likely that every patient develops at least a small perirenal hematoma.

- The mean fall in hemoglobin after a percutaneous kidney biopsy is 1 g/dL.
- Gross hematuria occurs in 2% of the cases and may require prolonged bed rest, bladder irrigation, and possibly evacuation of clots by cystoscopy.
- About 1% of patients will require blood transfusions.
- Prolonged and severe hemorrhage can be controlled with angiographic embolization of the bleeding vessel.

4.2　Introduction to Glomerular Disorders

(N Engl J Med 1998;339:888)

Introduction: Glomerular disorders have a variety of presentations and clinical courses that are related to the pattern of glomerular injury. They are traditionally classified by the manifestations of disease that are seen in their classic presentations; however, this classification is limited in clinical practice due to substantial overlap among the disorders and their presentations. This is further complicated by the evolution of patterns over time. Common clinical presentations of glomerular disease are discussed below followed by a discussion of individual glomerular disorders.

Asymptomatic Microscopic Hematuria

Cause:
- Urological diseases that are beyond the scope of this book
- IgA nephropathy (see Chapter 4.10)
- Thin basement membrane disease (see Chapter 4.18)

Epidem: IgA nephropathy and thin basement membrane disease can present at any age.

Pathophys: Disruption of the glomerular basement membrane or mesangial region

Crs: These glomerular disorders have a good prognosis.

Cmplc: Loss of kidney function, development of proteinuria

Lab: RBC casts, dysmorphic RBCs. UTI should be excluded. If proteinuria is present, the likelihood that the hematuria is glomerular and not urological is increased. The exact diagnosis can be made with a kidney biopsy, but it should rarely be performed in this setting because of the generally good prognosis of these conditions.

Xray: Kidney imaging with CT or US is needed to exclude tumors, polycystic kidney disease, stones, or other anatomic abnormalities. Individuals over the age of 40 should have a cystoscopy to rule out urothelial cancer.

Rx: Usually not needed given the good prognosis

Asymptomatic Gross Hematuria

(Am Fam Physician 2005;71:1949)

Cause:

- Urological diseases that are beyond the scope of this book
- IgA nephropathy
- Postinfectious, particularly poststreptococcal, GN (see Chapter 3.3)

Epidem: Both IgA nephropathy with episodic gross hematuria and postinfectious glomerulonephritis are seen in children.

Pathophys: Disruption of the mesangial lesion occurs in IgA nephropathy while postinfectious glomerulonephritis involves active glomerular inflammation.

Sx: Flank pain may be present.

The timing of pharyngitis and the onset of hematuria can help distinguish these disorders.

- In IgA nephropathy, the onset of hematuria is within a day of the onset of a sore throat.
- In postinfectious glomerulonephritis, there is usually a 2–3 wk delay between the respiratory infection and the onset of hematuria.

Crs: Hematuria is recurrent in IgA nephropathy. While most patients with poststreptococcal glomerulonephritis will recover spontaneously, they may have persistent microscopic hematuria for a prolonged period.

Cmplc: Severe presentations of poststreptococcal GN with renal failure requiring dialysis or difficult to control hypertension

Lab: Postinfectious GN will usually present with proteinuria and low complement (particularly low C3). ASO titers peak about 4 wk after the invasive streptococcal infection.

Xray: Imaging is useful in excluding urological disease.

Rx: Discussed in individual disease sections.

Benign Orthostatic Proteinuria

(Adolesc Med Clin 2005;16:163)

Cause: A condition of children or adolescents where abnormal protein excretion occurs only when the subject is upright.

Epidem: This condition is only seen in children or adolescents. Adults should not be worked up for this condition.

Pathophys: Poorly understood

Crs: Benign long-term prognosis

Lab: Proteinuria on routine dipstick urinalysis. A morning urine specimen collected after a full night of being supine with a protein to creatinine ratio of 0.2 or less is consistent with this diagnosis in a pediatric patient. A split 24-hr urine collection, with the urine collected after being supine placed in a separate container, should be collected. If this collection demonstrates normal urinary protein excretion while supine (urine protein to creatinine ratio of less than 0.150), then the presentation is consistent with benign orthostatic proteinuria.

Rx: No rx needed.

Asymptomatic Non-Nephrotic Proteinuria

(Clin Nephrol 1996;45:281; J Pediatr 1991;119:375)

Cause: Low-level proteinuria in individuals without history of renal injury and without history of chronic conditions that can cause proteinuria, such as diabetes or hypertension, is caused by glomerular disease of unknown cause.

Pathophys: Unknown glomerular injury. Biopsy will usually show a milder form of other well described glomerular diseases such as focal and segmental glomerulosclerosis, IgA nephropathy, or membranous nephropathy, which are discussed below.

Crs: Most patients will have a benign course and a good prognosis.

Cmplc: Progression to abnormal kidney function will occur in about 15% of patients.

Lab: Dipstick-positive proteinuria with a protein to creatinine ratio of less than 1 mg/dL protein per 1 mg/dL of creatinine or less than 1000 mg per 24 hr

Rx: No pharmacological rx necessary, but patients should be monitored for worsening proteinuria or development of hypertension or impaired GFR. In patients with progressive proteinuria, therapy with ACEIs or ARBs may prevent progression of the disease.

Nephrotic Syndrome

Introduction: Nephrotic syndrome is a condition that results from a specific pattern of glomerular injury, which changes the protein permeability of the glomerular structures and thus results in the development of proteinuria. It is characterized by the pentad of proteinuria of more than 3.5 g/d, hypoalbuminemia, edema, hypercholesterolemia, and lipiduria. Initially, the patients with idiopathic nephrotic syndrome will be normotensive and will have normal renal function. Usually they will have no cells or cellular casts in the urine. The list of common causes of nephrotic syndrome is shown in Table 4.1.

Table 4.1 Common Causes of Nephrotic Syndrome

Secondary Nephrotic Syndrome

Diabetic Nephropathy
Secondary FSGS
   Hypertensive nephrosclerosis
   Solitary kidney
   Reflux nephropathy
   Renal dysplasia
   Obesity
   Sickle cell disease
   Radiation nephritis
   Viral
      HIV
      Others
   Drug induced
      Heroin
      Pamidronate
Deposition Diseases
   Amyloidosis
   LCCD
Secondary Membranous Nephropathy
   Membranous lupus nephritis (class 5)
   Infections
      Hepatitis B
      Hepatitis C
   Drug induced
      NSAIDs
      Gold
   Malignancy
      Solid tumors

Idiopathic Nephrotic Syndrome

MCD
FSGS
Membranous nephropathy
MPGN

The site of injury in nephrotic syndrome involves the glomerular epithelial cell and the epithelial side of the basement membrane (Figure 4.1). Glomerular injury can be secondary to systemic conditions, such as diabetes mellitus or amyloidosis, or idiopathic conditions, such as MCD or FSGS. The nomenclature of these conditions can be confusing. A number of conditions are named for the pattern of injury as seen on light microscopy of the renal biopsy specimen. A pattern of injury with the same

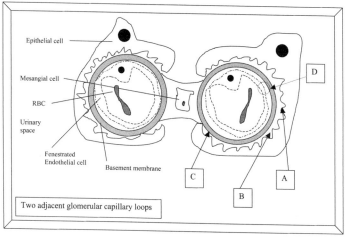

Epithelial cell

Mesangial cell

RBC

Urinary space

Fenestrated Endothelial cell

Basement membrane

D

C

A

B

Two adjacent glomerular capillary loops

Figure 4.1 Locations of Injury in Nephrotic Syndrome. Pathologic lesions that lead to the development of nephrotic syndrome typically involve fusion or effacement of epithelial cell foot processes (A), deposits on the subepithelial surface of the basement membrane seen in membranous nephropathy (B), and deposition of fibrils in immunoglobulin deposition diseases in the basement membrane and in the subepithelial space (B, C). Since the endothelial cell and the subendothelial space are not involved, hematuria is not seen in nephrotic syndrome (D).

name can be used to describe an idiopathic disorder or the consequences of secondary glomerular injury due to another condition. For example, the term FSGS is used as the name of an idiopathic disorder called *primary FSGS* and as the name of the lesion of hypertensive nephrosclerosis called *secondary FSGS due to hypertension.*

Prolonged sustained nephrotic syndrome can lead to a variety of complications, the most clinically important of which is progressive decline in kidney function. Not every patient with nephrotic range proteinuria will develop edema, hypoalbuminemia, or renal failure.

Common clinical consequences of the nephrotic syndrome include:

- Edema. The mechanisms of edema are related to low oncotic pressure and the poorly understood tendency for sodium retention by the nephron. Edema associated with the nephrotic syndrome is uncomfortable and should be treated with diuretics. This may predispose the patient to electrolyte disorders and intravascular volume depletion. Patients with nephrotic syndrome may be diuretic resistant due to the strong propensity for sodium retention and because filtered protein will bind the diuretic in the tubular space and will make it unable to act on its target receptor.
- Thrombotic complications more commonly include venous thrombosis and, rarely, arterial thrombosis. Renal vein thrombosis will complicate 20%–30% of cases of membranous nephropathy and may be asymptomatic. The cumulative incidence of thrombosis in nephrotic patients may be as high as 50%, which raises the question of prophylactic anticoagulation for all nephrotic patients (J Am Soc Nephrol 2007;18:2221). While venous thrombosis is predominant, the rate of coronary events is also increased.

- Hyperlipidemia is common and typically involves increases in VLDL and LDL while the HDL remains normal. There is currently a consensus that hyperlipidemia of nephrotic syndrome should be treated with lipid lowering agents to reduce the cardiovascular risk, particularly in patients in whom a rapid remission of the nephrotic syndrome is not expected.
- Acute kidney injury is sometimes seen with nephrotic syndrome. Patients are predisposed to AKI due to hypovolemia. This complication occurs most frequently with minimal change disease (Kidney Int 1993;44:638).
- Protein malnutrition is common. Nephrotic patients may lose 15% of the lean body mass, but the weight loss is often masked by the weight gain related to edema.
- Infection is now a less common complication of nephrotic syndrome than it has been in the past, but it is still seen. This susceptibility may be related to tissue disruption by edema and loss of antibodies in urine.

Rapidly Progressive Glomerulonephritis

RPGN is discussed in Chapter 3.3.

Nephritic Syndrome

Nephritic syndrome differs from nephrotic syndrome by the presence of inflammation within the glomerulus. The resulting inflammation may lead to renal failure, hypertension, hematuria, and proteinuria. Red cell casts and dysmorphic RBCs are pathognomonic of glomerular hematuria. Although the classic description of the nephritic state emphasizes lower levels of proteinuria, presentations of certain conditions can in fact be quite variable. In addition, disorders with similar patterns of injury may sometimes present as nephrotic or nephritic syndromes. Nephritic patients typically do not have a low albumin and tend to have edema due to renal failure rather than due to low albumin.

The pathologic lesion of nephritic syndrome involves glomerular hypercellularity due to an influx of inflammatory cells and glomerular cell proliferation. This can lead to the classic lobulated appearance of the glomerulus. Disruptions of the endothelial cell layer due to subendothelial deposits are seen along the endothelial side of the basement membrane, and duplication of the basement membrane may occur.

The common causes of nephritic syndrome are:

- Lupus nephritis
- IgA nephropathy
- Postinfectious glomerulonephritis
  - Poststreptococcal GN
  - Endocarditis
  - Visceral abscess
  - Shunt infection

Chronic glomerulonephritis is a traditional description of a disease state of CKD, hypertension, and abnormal urinalysis. Lupus nephritis is a classic example of the disorder of chronic glomerular inflammation leading to chronic loss of GFR.

4.3   Diabetic Nephropathy

(N Engl J Med 2002;346:1145; Am Fam Physician 2005;72:96)

Cause: Diabetes and insulin resistance

Epidem: Diabetic nephropathy is the most common cause of ESRD in the United States, Japan, and Europe. The incidence of diabetic nephropathy is increasing. Diabetic nephropathy will develop in as many as 40% of patients 15 yrs after the onset of type 1 diabetes. Some ethnic groups, such as Pima Indians, with type 2 diabetes are at a similar risk. On average, type 2 diabetes patients may be a bit less likely to develop diabetic kidney disease, but since the numbers of patients with type 2 diabetes are large, the majority of patients with diabetic kidney disease are type 2 diabetics. Diabetes is also the most common cause of the nephrotic syndrome.

Patients with proteinuric diabetic nephropathy have a dramatically increased risk of cardiovascular complications compared to diabetic patients without renal complications. This risk contributes to substantial excess mortality in this patient population. If progression to ESRD occurs, a diabetic on dialysis will have a 22% higher mortality rate than his nondiabetic counterpart at 1 yr and a 15% higher mortality at 5 yr.

Pathophys: The cause of renal injury in diabetes is poorly understood. Advanced glycosylation end products and oxidative stress may cause renal injury; in addition, microcirculatory changes within the kidney, such as hyperfiltration and increased renal plasma flow, may cause further injury.

Sx/Si: Early stages of diabetic nephropathy are asymptomatic. Since hypertension is nearly universal in diabetic kidney disease, signs and symptoms of severe hypertension can be seen in untreated subjects. If nephropathy progresses to nephrotic syndrome, edema and other complications of nephrosis may occur.

Crs: Diabetic nephropathy is usually a progressive disease. The initial hyperfiltration changes are silent. Eventually microalbuminuria (more than 30 mg of albumin per 1 g of creatinine), which is the first clinically detectable stage of the disease, develops. At this stage, the dipstick test for albuminuria is negative. Following the microalbuminuric stage, most patients will progress to overt proteinuria. Untreated patients may lose as much as 10 ml/min of GFR per yr. Progressive CKD and the development of nephrotic range proteinuria are common. Cardiovascular complications are a major source of morbidity and mortality.

Cmplc: Progression to ESRD, severe uncontrolled hypertension, complications of nephrotic syndrome, cardiovascular disease

Lab: At the time of diagnosis of type 2 diabetes, patients typically have had hyperglycemia for several years. For that reason, patients with the initial diagnosis of type 2 diabetes should be screened for renal disease with a dipstick urinalysis. If it is positive for protein, then overt proteinuria is present, and the next step is to quantify the urinary protein and creatinine with a spot urine protein to creatinine ratio or a 24-hr urine collection.

If overt proteinuria is not present, then annual screening for microalbuminuria with spot albumin to creatinine ratio should be initiated. The American Diabetes Association recommends 2 positive screening tests done within a 3-month period to establish a diagnosis of diabetic nephropathy. Since patients with type 1 diabetes usually have an abrupt onset of disease, the screening for nephropathy can be delayed for several years after the diagnosis of diabetes. Several circumstances can lead to a false positive screening test for albuminuria. These include strenuous exercise, high protein intake, or febrile illnesses.

When proteinuria is detected in a diabetic patient, one should not automatically assume that it is due to diabetic nephropathy, as an individual with diabetes can develop any of the disorders described in this chapter. The presence of diabetic retinopathy is highly predictive of the presence of diabetic kidney disease, and one can reasonably assume that a patient with diabetic retinopathy and albuminuria has diabetic kidney disease. If diabetic retinopathy is not present, a workup for other forms of proteinuric illness may be necessary. A kidney biopsy may be indicated in this setting. The presence of microscopic hematuria is not uncommon in diabetic kidney disease and does not exclude diabetic nephropathy.

Kidney Bx: The Kimmelstiel-Wilson lesion of nodular glomerulosclerosis is the classic lesion of diabetic nephropathy. This pattern of injury on renal biopsy is found in less than half of patients with diabetes. Diffuse thickening of capillary walls and mesangial expansion are seen more frequently. When this pattern is encountered on biopsy, the differential diagnosis should include monoclonal immunoglobulin deposition diseases. Immunofluorescence microscopy can help exclude those. Vascular disease, in particular hyalinization of the arteriolar walls, is frequently seen even in normotensive diabetic patients.

Rx: Meticulous glycemic control reduces the risk of new or progressive nephropathy in diabetic patients. Blood pressure control is critical for controlling proteinuria and for slowing the progression of the disease. ACEIs and ARBs reduce proteinuria and slow down the rate of loss of renal function in diabetic kidney disease. Because of interference with normal glomerular hemodynamics, a rise in serum creatinine is expected after the initiation of therapy. Caution is needed to avoid the initiation of these agents in volume-depleted individuals and in patients treated with NSAIDs. A 30% rise in serum creatinine is generally considered acceptable with initiation of an ACEI or an ARB. A more dramatic rise in serum creatinine should raise the suspicion of renovascular disease, which is relatively common in type 2 diabetics.

Dihydropyridine calcium channel blockers worsen proteinuria and may accelerate the progression of diabetic kidney disease. This effect is not observed when these agents are used in combination with ACEIs and ARBs. It is also not seen with the other classes of calcium channel blockers. The blood pressure goal of < 130/70 is currently considered to be optimal for patients with diabetic nephropathy.

Hyperkalemia is a risk of ACEI and ARB therapy. Given the beneficial effects of ACEI and ARB therapy, hyperkalemia can be managed with a low potassium diet and the addition of a loop or thiazide diuretic, which may be required for optimal blood pressure control.

Hyperlipidemia is common in diabetic patients with proteinuria. Treatment of hyperlipidemia with HMG-CoA reductase

GLOMERULAR DISEASES

inhibitors (statins) is known to decrease proteinuria and delay the progression of chronic kidney disease.

Tobacco smoking is a risk factor for the development and progression of diabetic kidney disease. Smoking cessation reduces the risk of progression of diabetic nephropathy.

4.4 Minimal Change Disease

(Clin J Am Soc Nephrol 2007;2:445)

Cause: Not completely understood phenomenon related to cell mediated immunity, which involves epithelial cell injury. In some cases, there is a clear association with NSAIDs, interferon, or Hodgkin's disease.

Epidem: MCD causes 90% of idiopathic nephrotic syndrome in children under age 10. It also causes about half of the cases of idiopathic nephrotic syndrome in older children but only 10%–15% of idiopathic nephrotic syndrome in adults.

Pathophys: It appears that there is a loss of charge of the basement membrane and injury to the foot processes of the epithelial cells.

Sx/Si: Rapid onset of edema with ascites and pleural effusions. Hyperlipidemia may lead to xanthomas. Hypertension may occur in adult patients, although it is rare in children.

Crs: At least 75% of patients will respond to initial therapy with steroids. In adults, time to response is longer than in children, who may respond as soon as in 2 wk. Some adults will require 4 months of steroid therapy to achieve a response. Relapse is very common, and most patients will relapse at least once. Approximately 25%–40% of the patients will experience frequent relapses. There are many cases of medication dependent patients who are unable to discontinue the drugs responsible for the induction of their remission. Progression to ESRD is rare and only occurs in treatment resistant patients.

Cmplc: Persistently nephrotic patients are at risk of the common complications of nephrosis discussed at the beginning of this section.

Lab: Normal renal function with hypoalbuminemia and hyperlipidemia is frequently seen.

Kidney Bx: The classic biopsy finding of completely normal appearing glomeruli on light microscopy and foot process effacement seen on electron microscopy

Rx: Daily oral steroids such as prednisone at 1 mg/kg or alternate day steroids 2 mg/kg are the usual first line therapy. Alternate day steroids may have a more favorable toxicodynamic profile, particularly with respect to cosmetic side effects. Slow tapers are usually undertaken once the remission is achieved. Patients taking prolonged steroid therapy should receive prophylaxis against peptic ulcer disease, particularly if they are simultaneously taking aspirin or other NSAIDs. Given the high risk of osteoporosis, prophylaxis and rx of osteoporosis may be appropriate.

The first relapse is usually treated with a repeat course of steroids, unless the patient is unable to tolerate them. Alternative second line agents include cyclosporine, cyclophosphamide, and MMF.

Cyclosporine achieves more rapid remissions than cyclophosphamide and causes rapid reduction in proteinuria as soon as it is started, but it is also more likely to lead to a relapse once it is discontinued. Cyclosporine dependence is common. Due to the substantial toxicities of cyclosporine and cyclophosphamide, there is growing interest in the use of MMF for a variety of glomerular disorders. In one publication, 5 out of 6 patients achieved a remission of MCD with MMF (Kidney Int 2002;61:1098). In another publication, the use of MMF in steroid-resistant children resulted in a substantial reduction in the need for steroids and also a reduction in relapse rates (Am J Kidney Dis 2003;42:1114).

4.5 Primary Focal Segmental Glomerulosclerosis

(Nephrol Dial Transplant 2004;19:2437; J Am Soc Nephrol 2004;15:2169)

Introduction: Several distinct histological variants of primary (idiopathic) FSGS have been recognized.

- Classic FSGS
- Cellular FSGS
- Tip lesion FSGS
- Collapsing glomerulopathy (also described as collapsing FSGS)

There may be important differences in the prognosis of these histologic variants. This section will discuss the idiopathic form of FSGS. Collapsing glomerulopathy and its subset, the HIV nephropathy variant, have dramatically different presentations, clinical courses, and prognoses. Collapsing glomerulopathy is discussed separately below.

Cause: FSGS is a form of glomerular epithelial cell disease caused by a poorly understood circulating factor present in the plasma of affected individuals. Individuals with this disease who progress to ESRD and receive a kidney transplant can develop nephrotic syndrome minutes after the implantation of the allograft. The nature of the circulating factor has not yet been characterized.

Epidem: The epidemiology of FSGS is the subject of several ongoing controversies. The number of cases of FSGS in the United States appears to be increasing. In the past, membranous nephropathy was the most common cause of idiopathic nephrotic syndrome in Caucasians; now FSGS is the most common cause of idiopathic nephrotic syndrome in both Caucasians and African Americans (Am J Kidney Dis 2004;44:815). This may not be true in other countries. FSGS is now the most common idiopathic glomerular disease that causes ESRD in the United States.

Pathophys: Poorly understood epithelial cell injury caused by an unknown circulating factor

Sx/Si: Edema

Crs: The ability to achieve a remission with treatment appears to be the same among the 3 groups of patients discussed in this section. The ability to respond to treatment depends on the severity of the involvement of the glomeruli by the scar. Tip lesion may have a slightly better prognosis. Patients with the cellular lesion present with heavier proteinuria but appear to have a similar prognosis once treated. Less than 50% of patients will achieve remission with treatment.

Spontaneous remissions of idiopathic FSGS are very rare, suggesting that rx is necessary in all patients. Patients who are able to achieve a remission with treatment are much less likely to have progressive loss of renal function and ESRD.

Recurrence after transplantation is common, and primary FSGS is the most likely idiopathic glomerular disease to recur after transplantation.

Cmplc: Hypertension and progressive renal failure in nonremitters are common. Persistently nephrotic patients are at risk of the common complications of nephrosis discussed at the beginning of this section.

Lab: Nephrotic range proteinuria that is often heavy, hyperlipidemia, and hypoalbuminemia are common at presentation.

Kidney Bx: Light microscopy will reveal segmental scars that can involve glomeruli to different degrees. Cellular lesion will demonstrate cellular proliferation, while the tip lesion will reveal an adherence of a single glomerular lobe to the origin of the proximal tubule.

Electron microscopy will reveal diffuse effacement of the epithelial foot processes. This finding is critical for differentiat-

GLOMERULAR DISEASES

ing between primary and secondary FSGS, which has important implications for how this disease is treated.

Rx: Prior to the initiation of immunosuppressive rx, it is important to ensure that a case of secondary FSGS not be treated with immunosuppression. Secondary FSGS is often possible to distinguish from the idiopathic form by a history of an inciting condition such as hypertension or reflux nephropathy (see Chapter 4.7). A diagnosis of secondary FSGS is also suggested by a history of gradual onset of subnephrotic proteinuria, and the biopsy will demonstrate focal effacement of epithelial cell foot processes that is often seen only in sclerotic areas in secondary FSGS.

Steroid therapy is the usual initial rx with 1 mg/kg of prednisone per day. In pediatric patients, remission is expected sooner than in adults. Adult patients should be prepared for an 8–12 wk course of full dose steroids that will be required to achieve remission. Appropriate prophylaxis should be considered, especially when it comes to osteoporosis.

Cyclosporine along with low-dose prednisone for patients who did not respond to steroids was evaluated in a randomized trial in which cyclosporine was adjusted to a total blood trough level of 125–225 mcg/L. After 26 wk of rx, 70% of the patients achieved complete or partial remission. Relapse was common, but the loss of renal function over time was slower in the treated group than in the placebo group (Kidney Int 1999;56:2220). Cyclosporine is often used as the second line rx for FSGS patients who fail to achieve a remission with prednisone. Cyclosporine is nephrotoxic and should be avoided in patients who present with substantial renal impairment or in those who have a lot of interstitial fibrosis on the initial renal biopsy. Cyclosporine with whole blood trough levels of 125–225 mcg/L is also an appropriate therapy for individuals who are unable to tolerate steroids.

Cyclophosphamide for FSGS has the best results for steroid dependency. It is generally not effective in patients who are unable to achieve a remission with steroids.

MMF has been tried in a number of small studies. In one publication, 44% of steroid resistant patients had a substantial reduction in proteinuria and preservation of renal function suggesting that MMF may be an appropriate treatment for steroid resistant patients (Clin Nephrol 2004;62:405).

Patients with persistent proteinuria and those with hypertension should be treated with ACEIs and ARBs for the purposes of reduction of proteinuria and blood pressure control.

4.6   Collapsing Glomerulopathy (Collapsing FSGS)

(Semin Nephrol 2003;23:209)

Cause: This disorder is considered to be a morphologic variant of FSGS and is believed to be caused by epithelial cell injury. This condition has unique associations with other conditions, such as HIV, and a unique prognosis and, therefore, is discussed separately from other forms of FSGS.

The most common cause of collapsing glomerulopathy is HIV infection. Idiopathic variants also exist. Collapsing FSGS also has been associated with pamidronate therapy, especially in patients with MM. Less frequent associations include interferon therapy and parvovirus B19 infection.

Epidem: The majority of cases of collapsing glomerulopathy is seen in HIV positive individuals. It appears that HAART is associated with reduced frequency of this complication.

Pathophys: Poorly understood but appears to involve direct injury to glomerular epithelial cells.

Sx/Si: Edema and symptoms of renal failure

Crs: At presentation, the disease tends to be very severe. Proteinuria of over 10 g/24 hr is common at presentation. While most patients with idiopathic FSGS present with preserved or mildly impaired renal function, collapsing glomerulopathy frequently presents with severe renal failure. Usually there is rapid progression to renal failure. HIV patients treated with HAART appear to have improved outcomes.

Cmplc: In addition to rapid progression to ESRD, all complications of nephrotic syndrome described above are common.

Lab: Heavy proteinuria, hyperlipidemia. HIV testing is mandatory for all individuals with nephrotic syndrome because this disorder is in the differential diagnosis of nephrotic syndrome.

Kidney Bx: Collapse of the entire glomerular tuft is seen instead of focal and segmental sclerosis.

Rx: Offending agents, such as pamidronate, should be discontinued. Treatment with prednisone may be attempted. HIV-positive patients should be treated with HAART.

4.7 Secondary Focal Segmental Glomerulosclerosis

(Nephrol Dial Transplant 1999;14 [suppl 3]:58)

Cause: Numerous renal insults may lead to the lesion of secondary FSGS. A detailed list of the causes of secondary FSGS is presented in Table 4.1. The insults that can lead to the development of the FSGS can be divided into several broad categories:

- Hemodynamic insults include conditions such as solitary kidney, renal dysplasia, hypertension, loss of functioning renal mass due to reflux nephropathy, obesity, renal transplant, and others.
- Immunologic renal injury such as the results of prior glomerulonephritis and interstitial nephritis.

- Agents such as NSAIDs, heroin, pamidronate, and radiation can induce nephrotoxic glomerular injury.
- Diabetic nodular glomerulosclerosis is discussed separately, but it can be classified as a form of nodular secondary glomerulosclerosis.
- HIV nephropathy discussed above is a form of FSGS secondary to HIV infection.

Epidem: Related to the underlying disorder

Pathophys: The path to glomerulosclerosis is different and depends on the individual causes of glomerulosclerosis. A variety of mediators and cell types can be involved.

Sx/Si: Depending on the degree of proteinuria and renal impairment, the disorder can be either asymptomatic, or it can present with symptoms of nephrotic syndrome or uremia and renal failure.

Crs: The clinical course depends on etiology and other factors. Since the term secondary FSGS is used to describe a variety of disorders, very different clinical courses can be seen. For example, collapsing FSGS due to heroin will inevitably lead to ESRD, while hemodynamically mediated secondary FSGS in the setting of obesity may have a relatively benign prognosis.

Cmplc: Worsening proteinuria and worsening renal function

Lab: Proteinuria is often subnephrotic (less than 3500 mg/24 hrs), particularly in patients with hemodynamically mediated secondary FSGS.

Rx: Meticulous control of hypertension and reduction of proteinuria with ACEIs and ARBs. Hyperlipidemia and diabetes should be treated if present.

4.8 Membranous Nephropathy

(J Am Soc Nephrol 2005;16:1188)

Cause: MN can be idiopathic or secondary to another condition. The list of causes of secondary MN is shown in Table 4.1. Idiopathic MN appears to be an autoimmune disease with the target antigen located on the glomerular epithelial cell.

Epidem: While there is still some debate as to whether MN or primary FSGS is the most common cause of idiopathic nephrotic syndrome, MN is certainly the most common cause of idiopathic nephrotic syndrome in older individuals. This disorder is unusual in children and usually presents in the 30s and 40s.

Pathophys: Poorly understood mechanism leads to formation of subepithelial deposits and proteinuria.

Sx/Si: Most patients develop uncomfortable edema. Since thrombosis and thromboembolism are common, a symptom of thrombosis, such as flank pain due to renal vein thrombosis, may be the presenting complaint.

Crs: There is substantial variability in the course of MN, particularly of the idiopathic form. About a third of the patients with idiopathic MN will have a spontaneous remission that usually occurs within the first 2 years after the diagnosis. The other two-thirds will either have persistent proteinuria without renal failure or will progress to renal impairment.

Rarely, patients with a previously stable nephrotic syndrome may develop crescentic glomerulonephritis.

Cmplc: All complications of nephrosis described above can occur. For unknown reasons, patients with this condition are prone to renal vein thrombosis.

Lab: Proteinuria, hyperlipidemia, and hypoalbuminemia are typical in nephrotic syndrome. Laboratory workup is required to exclude secondary causes (ANA, C3, and C4 to exclude lupus nephritis and hepatitis B and C serologies).

Kidney Bx: Thickening of the capillary wall with characteristic "spikes," which are overgrowths of basement membrane around the immune deposits. Electron microscopy demonstrates subepithelial electron dense deposits that parallel the appearance of the IgG-stained deposits on the immunofluorescence microscopy.

Xray: While the association between solid tumor malignancies and MN is well described, routine scanning for cancer beyond what is needed for routine medical care is not the customary practice when MN is diagnosed.

Rx: As many as one-third of patients with MN will experience spontaneous remission during the first year after diagnosis. Thus observation for several months is appropriate for many patients. Those with a lower level of proteinuria, normal kidney function, and younger patients are likely to have a spontaneous remission and do not require immediate initiation of therapy. Patients with proteinuria of less than 4 g/d and normal renal function can be treated with BP control, ACEI, and ARBs.

Patients with heavier proteinuria or progressive disease should be treated with immunosuppressive therapy in addition to the above measures. The regimen described by Ponticelli used alternating months of steroids and chlorambucil and produced a significant improvement in renal survival (Kidney Int 1995;48:1600). Chlorambucil is no longer commonly used. More recently, a similar approach using cyclophosphamide has been utilized. Patients were treated with cyclophosphamide at 2.5 mg/kg/d during months 2, 4, and 6. Methylprednisolone iv was given in pulses of 1 g/d for 3 d at the beginning of months 1, 3, and 5 followed by oral prednisone 0.5 mg/kg/d for the remainder of these months (J Am Soc Nephrol 1998;9:444). In patients with some degree of renal impairment, daily oral cyclophosphamide at 1.5–2.0 mg/kg/d along with methylprednisolone iv given in pulses of 1 g/d for 3 d at the beginning of months 1, 3, and 5 followed by oral prednisone at 0.5 mg/kg every other day was given. The treatment was continued for 6 months and proved effective, but a high relapse rate was observed (Nephrol Dial Transplant 2004;19:1142).

Cyclosporine has also been studied as an agent for the treatment of idiopathic MN. It was effective in a manner similar to that of the above-mentioned regimens. A high rate of relapse was seen with this agent as well (Kidney Int 2001;59:1484).

There is experience with MMF therapy in MN. MMF at 1000 mg twice a day resulted in a remission in 66% of patients, whereas historical controls had a 72% remission rate with a cytotoxic regimen (Am J Kidney Dis 2007;50:248). This may be a promising agent, but the randomized trials have yet to be conducted.

Rituximab and eculizumab have shown promise in the treatment of MN, but larger series are needed prior to widely recommending these therapies.

4.9 Membranoproliferative Glomerulonephritis

(Nephrol Dial Transplant 2001;16[suppl 6]:71)

Introduction: MPGN is a pattern of glomerular injury seen in the biopsy specimens and not a specific disorder. MPGN can be idiopathic or secondary to another condition. In many cases, MPGN pattern of injury results from formation and then glomerular deposition of circulating immune complexes within the glomerulus that is then followed by inflammation. Idiopathic MPGN is more common in children. In adults, most cases of MPGN today are due to hepatitis C infection. Three distinct types of MPGN are recognized. Type I can be idiopathic or secondary to a number of infectious or autoimmune conditions. Type II MPGN, also called *dense deposit disease*, is a very rare idiopathic disease of children, due to uncontrolled activation of the alternative complement pathway. Type III MPGN is characterized by the blending of features of MPGN with those of membranous nephropathy and is usually due to hepatitis B or C.

Idiopathic Membranoproliferative Glomerulonephritis

(J Am Soc Nephrol 2005;16:1392; Nephrol Dial Transplant 2001;16 Suppl 6:71)

Cause: Unknown. Many cases are associated with nephritic factors, which are autoantibodies that can induce complement activation.

Epidem: Idiopathic MPGN is seen mostly in children.

Pathophys: Glomerular inflammation due to trapping of immune complexes in the subendothelial space

Sx/Si: Idiopathic MPGN usually presents as nephrotic syndrome in children. It can present with a more nephritic picture with proteinuria, hematuria, and hypertension. Children with type II MPGN will also often have loss of vision.

Crs: Idiopathic MPGN has a poor prognosis, and progression to ESRD is common.

Cmplc: Complications of nephrotic syndrome discussed above and renal failure.

Lab: Hypocomplementemia is usually seen. In type I MPGN, the classical pathway of complement will be activated with normal (sometimes low) C3 and a low C4. In type II MPGN, the alternative pathway is active, and C3 is low while C4 is normal.

When MPGN pattern of injury is observed, a search for a secondary cause is mandatory, particularly in an adult. Hepatitis B and C serologies should be obtained, and HIV needs to be ruled out. Lupus nephritis should be excluded with an ANA and anti-DNA antibodies. Cryoglobulinemia should be ruled out along with chronic bacterial infections, particularly endocarditis.

Kidney Bx: The glomeruli of MPGN patients are hypercellular due to influx of inflammatory cells and proliferation of glomerular cells. Sometimes hypercellular glomeruli are described as lobular in appearance. Double contoured capillary walls, also called *tram tracks*, are common. Variable deposition of IgM, IgG, and C3 is seen on immunofluorescence microscopy.

Several conditions have the appearance of tram tracking but are very distinct from the pathophysiology perspective. These include:

- TTP, HUS, and other thrombotic microangiopathies
- Antiphospholipid antibody syndrome
- Scleroderma renal damage and malignant hypertension
- Radiation nephropathy
- Sickle cell nephropathy
- Fibrillary glomerulonephritis
- Chronic transplant glomerulopathy

The absence of subendothelial deposits on electron microscopy should help distinguish between these conditions and MPGN.

Rx: Various immunosuppressive strategies, as well as treatments with aspirin and dipyridamole, have been tried with limited success.

Secondary Membranoproliferative Glomerulonephritis

(N Engl J Med 1993;328:465)

Cause: The most common cause of secondary MPGN of both type I and type III is cryoglobulinemia caused by hepatitis C. Other causes include other forms of cryoglobulinemia, chronic hepatitis B, endocarditis, dental or visceral abscess, chronic liver disease, and autoimmune diseases such as systemic lupus and hematological malignancies, particularly CLL.

Epidem: Since hepatitis C may cause as much as 80% of secondary MPGN, the epidemiology of MPGN will relate to the local epidemiology of hepatitis and other infections.

Pathophys: Circulating immune complexes and cryoglobulin-containing antigens are trapped in the glomeruli where they set off an inflammatory response.

Cryoglobulins are classified into 3 categories (Blood Rev 2007;21:183):

- Type I cryoglobulins are monoclonal IgGs, IgMs, or IgAs. Type I cryoglobulinemia is produced by hematological malignancies that produce monoclonal immunoglobulins. These include MM, Waldenstrom's macroglobulinemia, and other B cell disorders.
- Type II (mixed) cryoglobulins are polyclonal IgG and monoclonal IgM. These can be seen in hepatitis C, essential cryoglobulinemia, and CLL. Why hepatitis C leads to production of a monoclonal IgM is incompletely understood and may be related to the infection of a single B cell clone by the hepatitis C virus. This monoclonal IgM has rheumatoid factor activity.
- Type III (mixed) cryoglobulins are polyclonal IgG and polyclonal IgM. This disorder is associated with hepatitis B or C, essential cryoglobulinemia, a number of autoimmune conditions, and a number of bacterial, viral, and parasitic infections.

Sx/Si: Some patients will present with nephrotic syndrome while others will have a nephritic presentation. Rash (purpura) is common with cryoglobulinemia, along with weakness and arthralgias.

Crs: The outcome is usually poor unless an effective treatment is available.

Cmplc: In addition to progressive kidney dysfunction, cryoglobulinemic vasculitis may involve other organs where it can cause ischemia.

Lab: There are 2 clinical scenarios one is likely to encounter during an MPGN workup:

- Presentation with nephrotic or nephritic picture, where MPGN is a part of the differential diagnosis. In this situation, an extensive serologic workup of GN is appropriate, as described in the section on approach to the patient with glomerular disease. Given that idiopathic MPGN is less common than the secondary form, the workup should aim to exclude the infectious or autoimmune conditions that are commonly associated with secondary forms of MPGN.
- In a situation where an MPGN pattern of injury has been discovered in a kidney biopsy specimen, 2 critical issues need to be addressed:
  1. If this is the MPGN pattern of injury where neither true glomerular inflammation nor hypocomplementemia is present, then the differential diagnosis includes:
     - TTP, HUS, and other thrombotic microangiopathies
     - Antiphospholipid antibody syndrome
     - Scleroderma renal damage and malignant hypertension
     - Radiation nephropathy
     - Sickle cell nephropathy
     - Fibrillary glomerulonephritis
     - Chronic transplant glomerulopathy
  2. Once the above conditions that are associated with the MPGN pattern of injury but without glomerular inflammation have been excluded, a thorough workup for the much more common secondary causes of MPGN should be undertaken with the following laboratory testing:
     - Measurement of complement levels because hypocomplementemia will help confirm the presence of an immune complex disease.
     - Serologic, virologic, and microbiologic testing for conditions known to cause secondary forms of MPGN. In

patients with biopsy proven MPGN, hepatitis C should be definitively ruled out with a viral load if the serology is negative. HIV testing and hepatitis B serologies should be performed. Blood cultures are frequently overlooked in afebrile patients, but a number of low-grade infections (not just endocarditis and shunt infections) can cause MPGN. Diabetics in particular should be considered at high risk of chronic low-grade infections such as those of the diabetic foot.

- Autoimmune disease, particularly systemic lupus, should be excluded with ANA and anti-DNA antibody measurements.
- Screening for cryoglobulinemia and monoclonal light chains is necessary.

Rx: Since hepatitis C causes the vast majority of secondary MPGN cases, treatment of hepatitis C with pegylated interferon and ribavirin is central to the rx of MPGN secondary to hepatitis C. In cases of severe cryoglobulinemia with RPGN or vasculitis of vital organs such as the lung or ischemia of the digits, an aggressive immunosuppressive rx is required. Pulse iv methylprednisolone along with cyclophosphamide and possibly plasma exchange is required to control the life-threatening disease. Once control of the life-threatening manifestations of the vasculitis is established, specific therapy for hepatitis C can be initiated.

4.10   IgA Nephropathy

(N Engl J Med 2002;347:738; Clin J Am Soc Nephrol 2007;2:1054)

Introduction: IgA nephropathy is the most common form of primary glomerulonephritis in the world. It is a specific form of immune complex glomerulonephritis, and primary and secondary forms of this disorder have been recognized. This disease has a variety of presentations and a great variability of clinical course. Crescentic IgA nephropathy and its systemic variant Henoch-Schönlein purpura are an important cause of RPGN.

Cause: The cause of the primary form of IgA nephropathy is unknown. See Figure 3.1 for mechanism of crescent formation. Secondary causes include:

- Liver disease (cirrhosis, alcoholic hepatitis)
- Gastrointestinal disease (celiac sprue and inflammatory bowel disease)
- Autoimmune diseases (psoriatic arthritis and ankylosing spondylitis)

Epidem: Epidemiology of IgA nephropathy varies by region. In Japan and Korea, IgA nephropathy is responsible for nearly 50% of all cases of glomerulonephritis. In Japan, 40% of all cases of ESRD are caused by IgA nephropathy. This disease is more common in whites than in blacks. There is a male predominance of this disease. In Japan, the male to female ratio is 2:1. In the United States and northern Europe, it may be as high as 6:1. Familial clusters of this condition have been reported, but the disorder is sporadic in the vast majority of cases. The incidence of this disease is approximately 5–40 new cases per million of population per year.

Pathophys: IgA nephropathy is a systemic disorder with a poorly understood mechanism. Transplantation of a kidney from one individual with mild IgA nephropathy to another individual without IgA nephropathy led to rapid resolution of the IgA deposits in the transplanted kidney; this suggests that IgA nephropathy is a systemic disease. Abnormal glycosylation of IgA and the presence of anti-IgA IgG antibodies have been proposed as the possible mechanisms of this disorder.

Sx: Many patients with IgA nephropathy are completely asymptomatic, and the disease may be recognized as a result of routine screening or medical care of other conditions. Some patients will present with a classic symptom of gross hematuria (tea-colored urine without clots) that begins at the same time as a respiratory infection. About 20% of patients present with well established severe renal impairment and symptoms of uremia and hypertension.

Crs: The clinical course of IgA nephropathy is highly variable. Many patients will have a benign course, while others will progress to CKD and ESRD. The rate of progression to ESRD has been reported to be between 15%–40% over a lifetime.

Rapidly progressive crescentic disease is rare, particularly in adults, but it should be considered in the differential diagnosis of RPGN. Several indicators have been suggested as signaling a poor renal prognosis:

- Persistent microscopic hematuria
- Persistent proteinuria of more than 1 g per 24 hr.
- Hypertension
- Impaired kidney function at presentation
- High glomerular histopathological scores

Cmplc: Progression to ESRD and complications of the nephrotic syndrome described above for patients with nephrotic range proteinuria.

Lab: Some patients will have elevated serum levels of IgA, but these are not present in all cases and are neither sensitive nor specific. A patient presenting with microscopic hematuria, proteinuria, and other manifestations of glomerular disease should undergo a complete workup as described in the approach to the patient with glomerular disease section.

Kidney Bx: IgA nephropathy can only be diagnosed with a kidney biopsy. A wide variety of glomerular lesions can be seen. In the classic presentation of this condition, there are mesangial expansion and mesangial IgA deposits. Mesangial hypercellularity is also present. Other light microscopy lesions include diffuse endocapillary proliferation. Segmental sclerosis, necrosis, or crescent formation can also be seen. All the same light microscopy findings are commonly seen in a number of other conditions, thus it is critical to identify IgA deposits by the immunofluorescence microscopy. These deposits appear electron dense on electron microscopy. There may be a poor correlation between the severity of the histological disease and clinical presentation.

Rx: Crescentic IgA nephropathy, particularly the cases that present as RPGN, should be treated with steroids along with alkylating agents. Pulses of 1000 mg of methylprednisolone combined with oral cyclophosphamide at 1.5 mg/kg/d for 3 months are recommended for crescentic disease. Several small studies demonstrated improved outcomes with this aggressive approach to rx of crescentic proliferative disease.

For patients with nonproliferative disease who are likely to have a good prognosis (isolated intermittent microscopic hematuria with no hypertension and minimal proteinuria), no treatment is necessary.

Patients who are hypertensive and those who present with significant proteinuria and hypertension should be treated with an ACEI or ARB. The magnitude of benefit related to the use of these agents is not clear, but they do lead to an improvement in proteinuria and hypertension, which are both risk factors for progressive disease.

The use of omega-3 fish oil supplements is believed to be beneficial, although there is some conflicting data. Given the safety of this therapy, it is reasonable to recommend it to patients with IgA nephropathy who have risk factors for progression. This treatment may not be effective in individuals with proliferative forms of IgA nephropathy.

Steroid therapy has been studied in a variety of patients with IgA nephropathy. In nonproliferative forms of disease, steroid therapy may reduce proteinuria but is probably not effective in prolonging renal survival. In proliferative forms of renal disease, steroids do reduce proteinuria and may contribute to preservation of renal function.

MMF has been tried in a few small trials, but there is no sufficient data to recommend its use in IgA nephropathy.

Tonsillectomy is a popular IgA nephropathy treatment in some countries. The use of tonsillectomy is best reserved for the patients with recurrent episodes of pharyngitis accompanied by gross hematuria.

Renal transplantation is an excellent treatment for patients with IgA nephropathy who progress to ESRD. The recurrence rate of IgA nephropathy in renal allografts is 20%–60%. IgA nephropathy recurring in the allograft does accelerate graft loss in about 15% of patients who have recurrence. Recurrence of IgA nephropathy is equally likely to occur in grafts from related and unrelated donors, and transplantation from closely related donors should not be discouraged.

4.11   Systemic Lupus Erythematosus Nephritis

(J Am Soc Nephrol 2004;15:241; Clin J Am Soc Nephrol 2006;1:863)

Cause: SLE is a systemic autoimmune disease of which the cause is incompletely understood. SLE involves development of various autoantibodies and dysregulated apoptosis of the immune system. The classic autoimmune phenomenon in SLE is the development of antibodies directed against DNA; however, many more autoimmune responses are also seen in SLE patients.

Epidem: SLE is much more common in women than in men. Not all patients with SLE will develop nephritis. Lupus nephritis is more common in African Americans and in pediatric patients with SLE.

Pathophys: A variety of mechanisms are involved in the pathogenesis of SLE nephritis. Antibodies, trapping of immune complexes, and other mechanisms of autoimmune toxicity injure the kidney. Antiphospholipid antibodies and cryoglobulins can also contribute to glomerular injury. A TMA such as TTP may produce its own form of glomerular damage. Finally, a subgroup of SLE patients has been found to produce ANCA. These patients may be subject to tissue injury by the same poorly understood mechanisms seen in ANCA vasculitis (see Chapter 3.3).

Si/Sx: Patients with SLE often have a variety of extrarenal manifestations that are much more symptomatic than renal disease. In the early stages of disease, particularly if renal function is preserved, the renal lesions may be completely asymptomatic.

Patients with the membranous renal lesion may develop various manifestations of nephrotic syndrome.

Crs: Lupus nephritis is a chronic disease. The course of this condition is closely related to the pattern of glomerular lesion seen on the initial biopsy as well as the amount of damage seen after 6 months of therapy. Patients with crescentic disease and those with extensive involvement of multiple glomeruli do worse. A lot of interstitial fibrosis on the initial biopsy is also a bad prognostic factor.

Cmplc: Numerous complications of SLE have been described that are related to the rx as well as the disease itself. From the renal standpoint, progression to CKD and ESRD are the most feared complications.

Lab: Positive ANA and antibodies against other nuclear antigens, such as Sm, Ro and La, will be present. Low complements will be noted. In cases of TMA and autoimmune hemolytic anemia, elevated LDH and undetectable haptoglobin can be seen.

Kidney Bx: The World Health Organization (WHO) first developed the classification of lupus nephritis pathology in the 1970s, and the classification has been modified subsequently. This system is in wide use today, and additional modifications have been proposed. An additional system has been developed to score the activity of inflammation and the chronicity of the damage. Activity is graded with a score of 0–24, and chronicity is graded on a scale from 1 to 12. Tubuloreticular inclusions are a classic finding in the endothelial cells of the kidney biopsy specimens of patients with lupus nephritis. These form in response to inflammatory cytokines and can be helpful in distinguishing lupus nephritis from other forms of glomerular disease. Some patients have a predominantly vascular pattern of injury that may be related to a TMA or an antiphospholipid antibody syndrome. Some patients have only interstitial nephritis without any glomerulonephritis.

The WHO classification is widely used to guide rx and consists of 6 classes:

- Class I: Normal glomeruli but deposits can be seen on electron and immunofluorescence microscopy
- Class II: (a or b) Mesangial disease with 2 gradations of severity of mesangial expansion and hypercellularity
- Class III: (a, b, or c) With lesions of focal and segmental glomerulosclerosis. These are subclassified a-c based on the amount of necrosis and sclerosis.
- Class IV: (a, b, c, or d) Diffuse glomerulonephritis, which is also classified based on the presence of sclerosis or necrosis.
- Class V: (a, b, c, or d) Membranous glomerulonephritis with the pattern of injury similar to that of idiopathic membranous nephropathy. Classes Vb–Vd are used to describe the lesions that combine the features of the membranous nephropathy and those of lupus nephritis classes II–IV.
- Class VI: This class describes injury with advanced sclerosis where most glomeruli have severe irreversible damage.

Rx: Most of the literature regarding the rx of lupus nephritis centers on the treatment of patients with class III and class IV lupus nephritis. In those patients, monthly iv cyclophosphamide at 0.5–1 g/m^2 along with monthly iv methylprednisolone at 1 g/m^2 produces a remission approximately 85% of the time (Ann Intern Med 2001;135:248). This regimen has become the standard of care for proliferative lupus nephritis. This is usually followed by pulse iv cyclophosphamide every 3 months to maintain the remission. This regimen is associated with a significant amount of toxicity, such as the steroid side effects (infertility, ovarian failure, hair loss, cosmetic changes and avascular necrosis), as well as cyclophosphamide side effects (amenorrhea). Since so many lupus nephritis patients are young women, these side effects are of particular concern. Sensitivity regarding these side effects is required for the optimal care of lupus nephritis patients.

An approach with a shorter course of cyclophosphamide and steroids followed by azathioprine after 6 months of cyclophosphamide and steroid therapy was compared to the conventional therapy and produced similar results (Arthritis Rheum 2004;50:3934).

Cyclosporine can induce remission in patients who are refractory to other rx (Rheumatology [Oxford] 2000;39:218) or in those with the membranous pattern of injury (Lupus 2000;9:241).

MMF is effective for maintenance therapy after remission has been induced with steroids and cyclophosphamide but with a substantial reduction in toxicity, particularly infection (J Am Soc Nephrol 2005;16:1076). There is also evidence that induction therapy with MMF can be used as an initial therapy for proliferative or membranous lupus nephritis at least in the patients without overt renal failure at presentation (N Engl J Med 2005;353:2219).

Rituximab is a chimeric antibody against the CD 20. Rituximab causes depletion of CD 20 positive B cells, but it spares T lymphocytes. There is anecdotal information about the use of rituximab in SLE. Given the absence of randomized trials, this therapy should be reserved for patients resistant to other therapies or for those who have contraindications to the use of established therapies.

Pregnancy in patients with SLE in general and lupus nephritis in particular deserves special attention. The risk of fetal loss in women with lupus nephritis may be as high as 30%–40%. Women with lupus nephritis are also at risk of an unfavorable renal outcome such as progression to ESRD during or after the pregnancy. The presence of antiphospholipid antibodies dramatically increases the risk of an unfavorable fetal outcome as does heavy proteinuria and lack of remission of nephritis at the beginning of the pregnancy (Am J Kidney Dis 2002;40:713).

4.12 Kidney Disease Due to Antiphospholipid Antibodies

(Kidney Int 2002;62:733)

Cause: A variety of APLAs can cause renal disease. These can be associated with SLE or occur without any evidence of SLE. When APAs promote thrombosis in the absence of SLE, the condition is referred to as primary APAS.

Epidem: Inconsistent information is available regarding the presence of APLAs in SLE patients and their contribution to renal disease. Approximately one-third of lupus nephritis patients have some evidence of intraglomerular thrombosis due to APLAs. The pattern of renal injury in this setting resembles the pattern seen in TMA.

Pathophys: The pathophysiology of the APLA renal injury is poorly understood. It involves dysregulated coagulation, platelet activation, and endothelial injury.

GLOMERULAR DISEASES

Some patients tend to have arterial thrombotic events while others will have venous thrombosis or TMA. APLAs may also contribute to thrombosis of renal allografts. In the kidney, thrombosis of the large branches of the renal arteries, glomerular TMA, or renal vein thrombosis may occur.

Sx/Si: Given the large variety of renal and nonrenal manifestations of the APAs, a large variety of presentations ranging from deep venous thrombosis to stroke to pregnancy loss can occur as a result of this condition.

Lab: When involvement of the APLAs is suspected, the following workup should be undertaken:

1. Lupus anticoagulant assays: prolonged PTT due to the presence of an inhibitor of phospholipid dependent coagulation. The term *lupus anticoagulant* is a misnomer in 2 ways: (a) Many patients with this condition do not have SLE; (b) The anticoagulant effect is seen only in the PTT assay, while in vivo this condition is often associated with a hypercoagulable state. The inhibitor antibody prevents the correction of PTT when normal plasma is added. This enables one to differentiate this condition from clotting factor deficiency. Several lupus anticoagulant laboratory methodologies are available. The most sensitive test for the presence of lupus anticoagulant is the dilute Russell viper venom time.

2. Solid-phase ELISA assays for anticardiolipin antibodies and assays for antibodies against β2-GP1, which is a protein cofactor for antiphospholipid antibodies.

3. ELISA assays for other phospholipids

Caution is needed when interpreting these tests because antiphospholipid antibodies are seen in 3%–10% of asymptomatic individuals and can be present incidentally in other immune disorders such as post-infectious glomerulonephritis.

In cases of TMA, undetectable haptoglobin and elevated LDH along with schistocytes on the peripheral smear and thrombocytopenia will be seen.

Xray: The choice of imaging for the large artery or vein thrombosis should depend on the location of the suspected clot and local expertise. Angiography, duplex ultrasonography, CT angiography, MR angiography, and venography are available for confirming the diagnosis of an arterial or venous thrombosis.

Rx: The treatment for the antiphospholipid antibody-induced thrombosis is anticoagulation with warfarin to a goal INR of 3.5. Steroids decrease the titers of antiphospholipid antibodies but do not reduce the risk of thrombosis. There are anecdotal reports of the benefits of plasma exchange treatments in the antiphospholipid antibody-associated TMA, but the benefit is unclear.

4.13 Light Chain Deposition Disease

(Am J Kidney Dis 2003;42:1154; J Am Soc Nephrol 2006;17:2533)

Introduction: Light chain and heavy chain deposition diseases are glomerular disorders that result from the deposition of immune globulin fragments produced by a monoclonal population of plasma cells. In some cases, both light and heavy chains are deposited simultaneously. Isolated heavy chain deposition disease is a rare disorder that has unique features and is described separately below.

Cause: MM, B cell lymphoma, Waldenström macroglobulinemia, or a condition with a population of monoclonal plasma cells that does not meet all of the criteria for the diagnosis of MM

Epidem: MM and related conditions occur in older adults.

Pathophys: Deposition of monoclonal immune globulin (Ig) chain fragments in the glomerular basement membrane. In more than

70% of cases, kappa light chains form the deposits that lead to epithelial cell injury and nephrotic syndrome. This condition often coexists with cast nephropathy. In about 10% of cases, simultaneous deposition of light and heavy chains occurs. Hypertension and renal failure are common. In addition to the kidneys, light chain deposits can also be seen in the myocardium, hepatic, and neural tissues.

Sx/Si: Related to nephrotic syndrome, renal failure, and MM

Crs: Most patients present with MM and renal involvement at the same time. Usually, renal function is impaired at presentation. Additional morbidity may be related to extra renal involvement, such as heart failure or hepatomegaly and portal hypertension. The median survival of patients with this condition is 4 yr. The majority of patients will progress to ESRD. Survival on dialysis is poor when myeloma is present.

Cmplc: When cast nephropathy is present along with LCDD, rapid progression to ESRD may occur. Recurrence in the allograft if transplant is performed is nearly universal.

Lab: The majority of patients will have monoclonal protein present on a serum or urine protein electrophoresis. A few patients will have no detectable monoclonal protein in serum or urine.

Kidney Bx: Light microscopy often reveals nodular glomerulosclerosis and diffuse thickening of the basement membranes, which can be similar in appearance to diabetic kidney disease. Thickening of the basement membranes of the tubules is also seen. Immunofluorescence demonstrates the light chain deposits, which are Congo red negative. Electron microscopy demonstrates granular deposits that do not form fibrils.

Rx: Chemotherapy and steroids, possibly with autologous stem cell transplant

4.14   Heavy Chain Deposition Disease

(Am J Kidney Dis 1999;33:954)

Cause: Plasma cell or B cell disorders with production of monoclonal immune globulin

Epidem: Plasma cell disorders, such as MM, are seen mostly in older adults. Most patients with heavy chain deposition disease do not have overt MM.

Pathophys: Isolated deposition of heavy chains is much less common than the light chain deposition disease. About 10% of patients with monoclonal immune globulin deposition diseases will have simultaneous light and heavy chain deposition. The defective heavy chains that are secreted in this condition can fix complement and cause low serum complement levels.

Sx/Si: Related to nephrotic syndrome, renal failure, and MM

Crs: Nephrotic syndrome with hypertension and loss of renal function

Cmplc: Progression to ESRD

Lab: Most patients with heavy chain deposition disease will have a monoclonal protein found in the blood, but that protein is usually not the heavy chain deposited in their glomeruli.

If the defective heavy chains are able to fix complement, low complements may be seen. Patients with heavy chain deposition disease often have a false-positive hepatitis C antibody test. The hepatitis C PCR test will be negative. This condition can easily be confused with membranoproliferative glomerulonephritis; both conditions will present with thickened basement membranes, low complements, and positive hepatitis C serologic tests.

Kidney Bx: Nodular deposits that may resemble the appearance of diabetic nephropathy as well as diffuse thickening of the basement membranes. On immunofluorescence, the heavy chains will be seen within the glomerular and tubular basement membranes.

deposits will be seen on electron microscopy as granu-
lot forming fibrils.

 otherapy and steroids, possibly with autologous stem cell
Rx transplant

4.15   Amyloidosis

(N Engl J Med 1997;337:898)

Introduction: Deposition of amyloid material in various organs causes
disruption that eventually leads to organ dysfunction. All
amyloid deposits share the ability to bind Congo red stain and
to form fibrils. Several disease processes can lead to the formation and deposition of amyloid fibrils. AL (primary) amyloidosis
is due to the production of monoclonal immune globulin light
chains that are able to form beta-pleated sheets. AA (secondary)
amyloidosis occurs as a result of chronic inflammatory conditions,
which can be autoimmune or infectious in nature. There are also
less common familial forms of amyloidosis. The most common
form of familial amyloidosis is due to a transthyretin mutation.
This condition is not associated with nephrotic syndrome and
has mostly neurological manifestations. Other less common forms
of familial amyloidosis can cause nephrotic syndrome.

AL Amyloidosis (Primary Amyloidosis)

(J Am Soc Nephrol 2006;17:2533; Kidney Int 2002;61:1)

Cause: MM, B cell lymphoma, Waldenström macroglobulinemia, or a
condition with a population of monoclonal plasma cells that does
not meet all of the criteria for the diagnosis of MM

Epidem: Amyloidosis and MM are diseases of older adults. AL amyloidosis is more common in men than in women. Up to 30% of
patients presenting with MM have amyloidosis with variable
degrees of renal involvement. Only 20% of patients presenting

with AL amyloidosis will meet the criteria for the diagnosis of MM; most will have a milder plasma cell disorder.

Pathophys: Immune globulin light chains (usually lambda light chains) that are able to form beta-pleated sheets and aggregate into fibrils that deposit in the kidneys, heart, liver, peripheral nerves, and other tissues

Sx/Si: Given the broad range of possible organ involvement with amyloidosis, a variety of clinical presentations is possible. The predominant features will be related to the organ system with the most severe dysfunction. Patients with cardiac involvement may have signs and symptoms of heart failure, while those with neurological involvement will have symptoms of peripheral or autonomic neuropathy. Severe orthostatic hypotension is very common. Symptoms due to nephrotic syndrome and renal failure are common in the predominantly renal presentations. Macroglossia is the classic finding in patients with AL amyloidosis.

Crs: Poor outcomes are common in AL amyloidosis. Median survival is about 2 yr but can be even worse, particularly in patients with cardiac involvement. Nephrotic syndrome presentations with relentless azotemia are common, as are heart failure presentations.

Cmplc: Death, heart failure, and progression to ESRD

Lab: More than 90% of patients with AL amyloidosis have monoclonal light chains detected by the serum and urine protein electrophoresis and immunofixation. Lambda light chains are common in AL amyloidosis. An abdominal fat pad biopsy is usually the test of choice given its simplicity. Bone marrow biopsy is the reasonable second step, particularly as it may be indicated for the workup of possible myeloma. In patients with pronounced proteinuria, kidney biopsy will be diagnostic nearly 100% of the time.

Kidney Bx: Acellular deposits of the amyloid material in the glomeruli, blood vessels, and interstitium will be Congo red positive and will definitively establish the diagnosis. On electron microscopy, randomly arranged fibrils of 90–110 1 × 10⁻¹⁰ m are usually seen. Congo red positivity and deposits of fibrils will be identical in AL, AA, and familial amyloidosis.

    Immunofluorescence microscopy with fluorescent anti-lambda or anti-kappa antibodies may reveal the light chain that is causing the deposits. Lambda-light chains are more common than kappa in AL amyloidosis. The rate of false-negative immunofluorescence for the light chains is 35%; therefore, the absence of light chains in immunofluorescence does not exclude the diagnosis of AL amyloidosis, especially if a plasma cell disorder is evident on a bone marrow biopsy or if a monoclonal immune globulin is detected in urine or serum.

Rx: Patients with amyloidosis require supportive care for the involvement of various organ systems as well as attempts to control the production of the light chains by the malignant plasma cells.

    Supportive treatment for nephrotic syndrome includes diuretic and antihypertensive therapies. Heart disease requires specialized therapy by a cardiology consultant. Autonomic symptoms, particularly orthostatic hypotension, can be severe and extremely disabling. Treatment with compression stockings, fludrocortisone, and midodrine can be effective.

    Chemotherapy with prednisone, melphalan, and possibly an autologous stem cell transplant may benefit some patients with this condition. Because this tends to be a disease of older patients with significant comorbidities, most patients will not be fit for aggressive treatments such as autologous stem cell therapies.

AA Amyloidosis (Secondary Amyloidosis)

(N Engl J Med 1997;337:898)

Cause: Untreated inflammatory conditions (autoimmune or infectious). Rheumatoid arthritis, inflammatory bowel diseases, and familial Mediterranean fever are the more common autoimmune causes of this condition. Chronic persistent infections such as decubitus ulcer infections, bronchiectasis, or tuberculosis were once a common cause of AA amyloidosis.

Epidem: This is becoming a rare disease in the developed world due to the availability of better therapies for infectious and autoimmune diseases.

Pathophys: Serum amyloid proteins are formed as a result of inflammation. These acute phase reactants deposit in tissues in fibrils similar to other forms of amyloidosis.

Sx/Si: This condition presents as nephrotic syndrome with all of the typical manifestations. Macroglossia is not usually seen in AA amyloidosis.

Crs: The course and prognosis of AA amyloidosis depends on the outcome of treatment of the underlying disease. Involvement of the heart is rare; however, progressive renal deterioration can often occur.

Cmplc: Complications of nephrotic syndrome and loss of renal function

Lab: Since AL amyloidosis is much more common than AA amyloidosis, a workup is always necessary to rule out a monoclonal protein-producing plasma cell disorder with serum and urine protein electrophoresis.

Kidney Bx: Acellular deposits of the amyloid material in the glomeruli, blood vessels, and interstitium will be Congo red positive and will definitively establish the diagnosis. On electron microscopy, randomly arranged fibrils of 90–110 Å are usually seen. Congo red positivity and deposits of fibrils will be identical in AL, AA, and familial amyloidosis.

Rx: Treatment of the underlying disorder. Eprodisate is a compound that interferes with interaction between amylogenic proteins. Eprodisate has been shown to slow down the decline in renal function in AA amyloidosis (N Engl J Med 2007;356:2349).

4.16   Fibrillary Glomerulonephritis

(Kidney Int 1992;42:1401; Nephrol Dial Transplant 2004;19:2166)

Cause: Unknown

Epidem: This is a rare diagnosis seen mostly in adults. Fibrillary glomerulonephritis probably represents less than 1% of all cases of glomerular disease. Both genders appear to be equally affected.

Pathophys: Unknown

Sx/Si: Patients with this condition usually present with nonspecific symptoms of renal failure and proteinuria. Most patients will have nephrotic range proteinuria at presentation along with hypertension and microscopic hematuria.

Crs: Progression to ERSD over months to years is common.

Lab: Labs will be consistent with AKI or CKD and nephrotic syndrome. Monoclonal immune globulins are not present in the serum of patients with fibrillary glomerulonephritis.

Kidney Bx: Fibrillary glomerulonephritis can have a variety of light microscopic patterns. Membranous, membranoproliferative, and crescentic patterns may be seen. The diagnosis is made on electron microscopy that will demonstrate deposits of randomly arranged 20 nm fibrils.

Rx: There is no treatment that is proven effective for fibrillary glomerulonephritis.

4.17   Immunotactoid Glomerulonephritis

(Nephrol Dial Transplant 2004;19:2166)

Cause: Lymphoproliferative disorders are present in most cases before or after the diagnosis. Idiopathic cases have been described.

Epidem: This is a rare disease of older patients. This condition is seen in less than one-tenth of 1% of kidney biopsies.

Pathophys: Deposition of fibrils larger than those seen in fibrillary glomerulonephritis. Since many patients have monoclonal immune globulins associated with hematological malignancies, these deposits may be the precipitates of the immune globulins. These microscopic structures can organize into shapes resembling microtubules that are deposited in parallel rows. These structures are referred to as *tactoids*.

Sx/Si: Most patients will have findings consistent with nephrotic syndrome at presentation.

Crs: Most patients present with nephrotic syndrome and tend to have progressive loss of renal function. The patients' overall outcome may be related to their hematological disorder.

Lab: Many patients will have monoclonal immunoglobulin light chains detectable in serum or urine immune electrophoresis. Other abnormalities are related to hematologic malignancy and nephrotic syndrome.

Rx: Treatment of the underlying bone marrow disorder and supportive treatment for nephrotic syndrome and loss of kidney function

4.18   Diseases Due to Mutations of Type 4 Collagen

(Curr Opin Pediatr 2004;16:177)

Introduction: Mutations of the genes that encode different isoforms of type IV collagen can lead to hereditary nephritis (Alport Syndrome) and thin basement membrane nephropathy. In both of these conditions, a genetic defect leads to basement membrane abnormalities and hematuria. The principal difference between these conditions is the clinical course. Alport syndrome is associated with progressive kidney disease (particularly in males with the most common X-linked form of the disease), while thin basement membrane nephropathy tends to have a good prognosis. Traditionally, thin basement membrane nephropathy has been referred to as benign familial hematuria. While this description is generally true, it is now clear that some patients with thin basement membrane disease may develop progressive azotemia over time, and therefore the use of the word *benign* in the name of this condition should probably be avoided.

Hereditary Nephritis (Alport Syndrome)

(Curr Opin Pediatr 2004;16:177)

Cause: Mutation of one of several genes encoding alpha chains of type IV collagen.

Epidem: The most common form of this condition is X-linked. As a result, male patients tend to have the severe form of the condition. Since the genetic defect is present from birth, milder manifestations of this disease, such as hematuria, are present during childhood, while more severe manifestations, such as progressive azotemia, occur in older subjects.

Pathophys: Why thinning of basement membranes leads to progressive kidney disease is not completely understood. It is likely that uncontrolled deposition of some types of collagen on the subendothelial surface of the basement membrane leads to glomerular injury.

Sx: Some patients with this condition will develop hearing loss and an eye abnormality called *lenticonus* that leads to myopia.

Si: Anterior lenticonus is an anterior cone-shaped protrusion of the lens into the anterior chamber of the eye. While most patients with this condition do not have this finding, its presence is virtually pathognomonic of Alport syndrome.

Crs: Three distinct forms of Alport syndrome with different patterns of inheritance and different clinical features have been described.

- X-linked Alport syndrome is the most common form of the disease. It affects approximately 80% of the patients. Males with this condition have persistent microscopic hematuria. If hematuria does not appear by the age of 10, the disease is unlikely. Many affected males will also develop sensorineural deafness. Over time, affected males develop proteinuria (sometimes nephrotic range), hypertension, and progressive renal disease. Heterozygous female patients may have intermittent or persistent hematuria, and they are less likely to develop proteinuria or hypertension. Males (particularly those with hearing loss) are likely to have progressive disease, but the timing of development of ESRD is highly variable. Females are much less likely to develop ESRD. Members of some families develop leiomyomas of the respiratory system and the esophagus.
- The autosomal recessive form of this condition is much less common. Patients with this condition will not have the classic family history of affected males and relatively spared females. These patients have deafness and rapid progression to ESRD. This form of the disease should be suspected when a young female patient presents with hearing loss, hematuria, and proteinuria. When both copies of the defective gene are inherited by an individual and are not the result of a spontaneous mutation, it is likely that both of the affected individual's parents had thin basement nephropathy described below.
- Autosomal dominant Alport syndrome is a rare disorder, which has been described in several families with variable presentations.

Cmplc: Complications of nephrotic syndrome and progression to ESRD. Rarely, anterior lenticonus can lead to rupture of the lens capsule. Anterior lenticonus is associated with rapid progression to ESRD. About 90% of males with the X-linked disorder will develop deafness.

Lab: Genetic testing for this condition is not readily available. Hematuria with dysmorphic red blood cells and red blood cell casts can be intermittent early in the course of the disease making the presentation appear similar to IgA nephropathy.

Kidney Bx: Light microscopy will demonstrate a variety of patterns of injury. On electron microscopy, variable thickening and thinning of the basement membrane loops will occur in the same capillary loop. Basket weaving and lamellation of the basement membranes can also be seen.

Rx: There is no known effective treatment for the underlying defect in this condition. Treatment of hypertension and proteinuria with ACEIs and ARBs may retard the progression of renal disease. Treatment of other complications of the nephrotic syndrome, such as hyperlipidemia, may prevent complications in other organ systems.

Renal transplantation is an excellent treatment for patients with this condition who may be younger and will have fewer comorbidities than the majority of ESRD patients. A rare but significant complication of transplantation, which occurs in less than 5% of patients with Alport syndrome, is the development of anti-GBM disease in the allograft. This occurs due to the exposure of the transplant recipient's immune system to the normal type IV collagen and development of antibodies against it.

Thin Basement Membrane Nephropathy

(J Am Soc Nephrol 2006;17:813)

Cause: Inherited defect in the genes coding for some of the chains of type IV collagen

Epidem: Most of the cases of this condition go undiagnosed and their numbers unknown. While the disease has been reported mostly in the developed countries, this likely has to do with routine use of screening urinalysis. Thin basement membrane nephropathy is probably slightly more common in women than in men.

Pathophys: It is unclear why the defective collagen leads to hematuria and sometimes proteinuria.

Sx/Si: A small number of patients with this condition may occasionally have gross hematuria. One must keep in mind, however, that individuals presenting with gross hematuria after an infection or exertion are far more likely to have IgA nephropathy than thin basement membrane disease.

Crs: Usually benign and without progressive renal disease. Some patients may develop proteinuria and progressive renal impairment. It should be emphasized that there may be substantial difficulties in distinguishing this condition from Alport syndrome, even in patients who undergo a kidney biopsy, since the appearance of thin basement membranes will be the same in the early stages of Alport disease and in thin basement membrane nephropathy.

Lab: In order to be consistent with the diagnosis of thin basement membrane nephropathy, microscopic hematuria must be of glomerular origin (as evidenced by dysmorphic red cells or red cell casts) and persistent. A number of conditions, such as post-streptococcal glomerulonephritis, can lead to microscopic hematuria at some point. For that reason, individuals suspected of having thin basement membrane nephropathy should demonstrate glomerular hematuria on several occasions several years apart.

Kidney Bx: Light microscopy is close to normal with only occasional mesangial changes. Electron microscopy demonstrates thin basement membranes. There is currently a controversy as to the normal range of basement membrane thickness. Basement membranes that are less than 250 nm thick in adults probably constitute a thin basement membrane, but this issue requires care as a variety of pitfalls exist, such as differences in normal basement membrane thickness between genders. Special attention is required when interpreting biopsy specimens of children under 11 whose basement membranes grow in thickness as they age and, therefore, need to be examined in the context of the patient's age at the time of the biopsy. Thinning of the basement membranes seen in young subjects should be interpreted with caution as the differential diagnosis at that point includes both Alport syndrome and thin basement membrane nephropathy. Under these circumstances, a family history of progressive kidney disease and hearing loss may be very useful in making the correct diagnosis.

Rx: None needed.

Chapter 5

Inherited Kidney Diseases

5.1 Autosomal Dominant Polycystic Kidney Disease

(N Engl J Med 1993;329:332)

Cause: Almost all cases of ADPKD are due to either a mutation of the PKD1 gene on chromosome 16 or the PKD2 gene on chromosome 4. Autosomal dominant inheritance is responsible for 90% of cases, and the rest are due to a spontaneous mutation.

Epidem: ADPKD is the most common hereditary kidney disorder. It occurs at a rate of approximately 1/400 births and affects approximately 600 000 people in the United States and 12 million worldwide. It is the fourth leading cause of ESRD in the United States.

Pathophys: Increases in total kidney volume are associated with a decline in GFR (N Engl J Med 2006;354:2122). Cysts develop in a relatively small number of nephrons, but as the cysts enlarge, several changes take place in normal kidney tissue. These changes include regional tissue ischemia, interstitial fibrosis, inflammation, and cell death. The mechanisms responsible for cyst growth are *cellular proliferation* (large cysts have more cells rather than larger cells), fluid secretion, and extracellular matrix remodeling.

Sx: Pain, hematuria

Si: Increased abdominal girth, palpable kidneys, hypertension

Crs: Progressive loss of kidney function so that 50% of patients require dialysis or a transplant by the fifth decade of life. The median age at death or onset of dialysis is 53 years old for patients with the PKD1 genetic mutation compared to 69 years old for patients with the PKD2 mutation (Lancet 1999;353:103).

Cmplc:

- Kidney complications
  - Pain
  - Hematuria
  - Hypertension
  - Nephrolithiasis
  - CKD
- Extrarenal manifestations
  - Hepatic cysts
  - Colonic diverticula
  - Cardiac valvular abnormalities
  - Intracranial aneurysms

Lab: Genetic testing by DNA linkage analysis is available; it requires several affected and nonaffected family members. DNA sequence analysis can detect a mutation in 60%–80% of cases.

Xray: Abdominal ultrasound is the most commonly used test to diagnose the condition. In a patient with a family history of ADPKD, the presence of 3 or more cysts in each kidney by age 40 can establish the diagnosis. If there are no cysts by age 30, ADPKD is not present.

Patients with ADPKD who have a strong family history of intracranial aneurysms or headaches should be screened for intracranial aneurysms. MRA of the brain is a good screening test for this purpose.

Rx: Hypertension is associated with increased kidney size and worse cardiovascular outcomes (J Am Soc Nephrol 2001;12:194). A target blood pressure of less than 130/80 is recommended for patients with ADPKD. ACEIs or ARBs are a good choice in these patients due to activation of the renin-angiotensin system by regional ischemia within the kidney tissue.

5.2 Autosomal Recessive Polycystic Kidney Disease

(Pediatrics 2003;111:1072)

Cause: ARPKD is due to a mutation of the PKHD1 gene on chromosome 6.

Epidem: This is a rare disease inherited in an autosomal recessive pattern. It occurs in about 1/20 000 births. When both parents are carriers of the gene, there is a 1 in 4 chance the offspring will have the condition. There is usually no family history of the disease.

Pathophys: ARPKD is characterized by in utero development of cysts within the renal collecting tubules. Similar to ADPKD, cyst growth causes fibrosis, inflammation, regional ischemia, and cell death in normal kidney tissue. There are increased numbers of dilated and tortuous dilated bile ducts within hepatic tissue.

Si: Abdominal masses, Hypertension

Crs: 10%–30% of affected infants die as newborns. 80% of children who survive the first month will reach age 15 or greater.

Cmplc:

- Kidney
  - CKD
  - Hypertension
  - Abnormal concentrating ability
- Hepatic
  - Hepatic fibrosis
  - Portal hypertension
  - Acute bacterial cholangitis

Lab: Abnormal urinalysis, hyponatremia

Xray: Ultrasonography demonstrates enlarged kidneys that are diffusely echogenic. Antenatal diagnosis can be made as early as the 18th week of gestation (Prenat Diagn 1995;15:868).

Rx: Patients that survive infancy go on to develop progressive CKD. Hypertension, anemia, nutrition, and growth retardation often require extensive management during childhood. If patients go on to ESRD, they can be treated with dialysis or kidney transplantation. Some patients with severe hepatic involvement require liver transplantation.

5.3   Sickle Cell Nephropathy

(Am J Hematol 2000;63:205)

Cause: Sickle cell anemia and β-thalassemia

Epidem: The prevalence of the sickle cell gene is 8% in African Americans. It is as high as 25%–50% in some areas of Africa.

Pathophys: Sickle cell nephropathy is characterized by a defect in urinary concentrating capacity. This occurs because of ischemic damage to the inner renal medulla, which contains the long loops of Henle. Hypoxic conditions within the *vasa recta* (capillary network that supplies and drains the inner medulla) predispose erythrocytes to sickling and formation of thrombi, which in turn lead to infarctions within the deep medulla and sometimes papillary necrosis. Medullary infarction results in bleeding into the collecting system and hematuria. Loss of the deep medullary loops of Henle causes impairment in urinary concentrating ability. Individuals with sickle cell nephropathy are unable to achieve urine osmolality above 420 mOsm/L. Defects of urine acidification and potassium excretion can also be present.

Glomerular function is normal or supranormal at first. Over time, changes related to chronic hyperfiltration occur, and this may result in secondary FSGS.

Sx/Si: Hematuria, other manifestations of sickle cell disease

Crs: In the past, less than 30% of the patients were believed to develop proteinuria. In one recent series, microalbuminuria was seen in 42% of the patients. Overt proteinuria was seen in 26% of the patients. Nearly 70% of the patients with SS eventually developed evidence of glomerular disease. Less than 10% of the patients developed an overt renal impairment (J Am Soc Nephrol 2006;17:2228).

Cmplc: Hypertension, proteinuria, and impaired GFR

Lab: Screening for microalbuminuria appears to be appropriate for patients with sickle cell disease.

Rx: Patients with sickle cell nephropathy should avoid NSAIDs, which reduce medullary blood flow. It is not known at this time if treatment of proteinuria with ACEIs or ARBs will prevent loss of kidney function.

5.4 Fabry Disease

(J Am Soc Nephrol 2002;13[suppl 2]:S139)

Cause: Hereditary deficiency of the enzyme α-galactosidase A

Epidem: It is believed that there are between 1000 and 3500 males with this disease in the United States, and approximately 14 of them start dialysis every year.

Pathophys: The gene for the α-galactosidase A enzyme is located on the X chromosome. Multiorgan manifestations of the disease are much more severe in males. Tissue accumulation of the glycosphingolipid trihexosylceramide causes tissue damage in the kidneys, heart, skin, and nervous system.

Sx/Si: Angiokeratomas appear on the skin by the second decade of life. Shortness of breath can occur due to airway involvement. Autonomic and peripheral neuropathies are common, along with a variety of central nervous system manifestations, such as headache, ataxia, and problems with balance. Involvement of the coronary vessels leads to angina and myocardial infarction.

Crs: Untreated disease leads to death due to kidney, heart, or nervous system involvement.

Cmplc: A variety of complications in multiple body systems may occur. Prior to the availability of dialysis, death due to renal failure was the most common cause of death for patients with this disease. It usually occurred in the fourth decade of life.

Lab: Reduced serum levels of α-galactosidase A are diagnostic of Fabry disease. Patients with this disease usually present with proteinuria, hematuria, and CKD.

Kidney Bx: This disease produces vacuolization of the glomerular epithelial cells. Within those inclusions, electron microscopy reveals characteristic zebra bodies.

Rx: Aggressive treatment of hypertension and proteinuria with angiotensin blockade should be instituted for all patients with CKD.

Two recombinant preparations of α-galactosidase A, Fabrazyme and Replagal, are available. While long-term studies are yet to be conducted, it does appear that these preparations lead to improvement of glomerular architecture and possibly even renal function.

Hereditary Nephritis (Alport Syndrome)

See Chapter 4.18.

Thin Basement Membrane Nephropathy

See Chapter 4.18.

Inherited Causes of Hypokalemia

See Chapter 1.3.

Chapter 6

Tubulointerstitial Diseases

Introduction: Several kidney disorders involve inflammation and possible scarring of the renal interstitial space. While all disorders that lead to kidney failure involve progressive interstitial scarring, some conditions share the common feature of the interstitial compartment being the site of the initial injury. These include acute interstitial nephritis (AIN) (see Chapter 3.4) and chronic interstitial nephritis and reflux nephropathy (discussed below). Chronic interstitial scarring and fibrosis resulting from glomerular and systemic disorders is referred to as *secondary chronic interstitial nephritis*, while conditions where the interstitium is the site of primary injury are called *primary chronic interstitial nephritis*.

6.1   Primary Chronic Interstitial Nephritis

(Am J Kidney Dis 2005;46:560)

Cause: A wide variety of insults can lead to chronic interstitial nephritis. The complete list of the causes is shown in Table 6.1.

Table 6.1   Common Causes of Chronic Interstitial Nephritis

Drugs

Analgesics
  Phenacetin-containing compound analgesics
  NSAIDs
  Mesalamine

Table 6.1 (Continued)

Drugs

Medications

  Lithium

  Calcineurin inhibitors

      Cyclosporine

      Tacrolimus

  Antiviral medications

      Tenofovir

      Cidofovir

  Hematological disorders

      Light chain deposition disease

      Multiple myeloma

  Chinese herbs

      Aristocholic acid

  Heavy metals

      Lead

      Arsenic

      Cadmium

  Autoimmune diseases

      Systemic lupus erythematosus

      Sarcoidosis

      Sjögren's syndrome

      Inflammatory bowel disease

  Electrolyte disorders

      Chronic hypokalemia

      Chronic hypercalcemia

  Metabolic disorders

      Chronic urate nephropathy

      Hyperoxaluria

      Cystinosis

  Urological

      Pyelonephritis

      Urinary tract obstruction

      Balkan nephropathy

Epidem: CIN is a rare cause of ESRD in the United States; however, it is more common in other countries. Groups of individuals with a specific risk factor may be at a high risk of CIN with severe complications. For example, in the countries where compound analgesics containing phenacetin were popular, as much as a quarter of all patients developing ESRD in the 1960s and 1970s had analgesic nephropathy.

In lithium-related CIN, patients with the most severe impairments in renal concentrating ability and those with the longest duration of lithium therapy are the ones most at risk of developing progressive kidney disease.

Pathophys: Toxic and ischemic injury to the medulla is believed to be involved in the pathogenesis of CIN. Toxins can accumulate in the medulla due to the function of the countercurrent concentrating mechanism. This area of the kidney has low oxygen tension and a precarious vascular supply, both of which make it vulnerable to injury.

Sx/Si: Hypertension and si and sx of uremia

Crs: Usually a slow and progressive decline in kidney function

Cmplc: Progression to ESRD

Lab: Unlike in AIN, the urine sediment is bland and usually does not contain wbc or wbc casts.

Kidney Bx: The pathologic features of CIN are nonspecific. Interstitial fibrosis and tubular atrophy are features seen in most progressive kidney diseases.

Rx: Discontinuation of the offending agent and management of CKD

6.2   Reflux Nephropathy

(Postgrad Med J 2006;82:31)

Cause: Congenital abnormality of the vesicoureteral junction that allows the reflux of urine into the kidney. The defect is due to the inadequate length of the intravesical submucosal ureter. Infection in combination with reflux accelerates kidney damage.

Epidem: Some degree of vesicoureteric reflux occurs in 0.4%–2% of all healthy children. It is less common in black children. Many of the cases of reflux will resolve by age 2. Only a small number of children with vesicoureteric reflux will develop reflux nephropathy characterized by hypertension and CKD. During the first 6 months of life, reflux is more common in boys. After the age of 6 months, it is more common in girls. This condition can be inherited in an autosomal dominant manner. Reflux nephropathy is the most common cause of ESRD in children.

Pathophys: Sex differences in the mechanism of renal dysfunction in this condition exist:

- Most boys with this condition have congenital abnormalities of their kidneys in addition to reflux. Reflux is usually severe and can be detected antenatally or in infancy. In these patients, impaired kidney function is at least partly related to kidney dysplasia and hypoplasia.
- In females, the kidneys are more likely to be normal when the condition is first detected, and their reflux is less severe. Recurrent UTIs are common in these patients. Dysfunctional voiding exacerbates UTIs. Because these patients are more likely to be born with normal kidneys, their chances for renal preservation are better. The kidneys of these patients are often small and smooth and do not have focal scarring due to UTIs. It is not clear why vesicoureteric reflux predisposes to infection. Stasis of urine in various locations may play a role.

Sx: Some children will have loin pain, but most cases are asymptomatic when infection is not present. Frequent symptomatic UTIs will be seen in some patients. Children with vesicoureteral reflux commonly have nocturnal enuresis and dysfunctional voiding.

Crs: Given the differences in the pathophysiology of this condition between the sexes, 2 distinct patterns exist:

- Some patients (usually male) will develop hypertension and progressive CKD in childhood or early adulthood. These patients often do not have a history of recurrent UTIs and their renal failure and hypertension are likely related to renal dysplasia.
- Other (more commonly female) patients will have frequent UTIs, including frequent episodes of pyelonephritis. Progressive renal scarring can lead to the development of proteinuria and progressive CKD. This condition can be unilateral. Patients with unilateral reflux may develop hypertension without renal failure.

Cmplc: Complications of frequent infections as well as development of hypertension and ESRD

Lab: When proteinuria is present, it is a poor prognostic factor.

Xray: Diagnosis of vesicoureteric reflux can be made with several imaging methodologies:

- Voiding cystourethrography is most accurate for the diagnosis of reflux. This procedure is technically difficult and requires cooperation of the pediatric patients. Reflux commonly occurs intermittently and can be missed with this methodology. The filling of the ureter is graded according to the international classification of vesicoureteric reflux. Cystourethrography is not a good screening test for renal damage due to reflux.
- Ultrasound can be used to detect ureteral dilatation under a variety of circumstances, but it is highly operator dependent.

   The diagnosis of reflux nephropathy used to be made by iv urography when the disorder was first described. Radionuclide scanning with DMSA is widely used for demonstration of scarring that may be due to reflux. CT can also be used to demonstrate scarring due to pyelonephritis.

TUBULOINTERSTITIAL DISEASES

Rx: The goal of treatment in this condition is the prevention of kidney damage. Milder grades of reflux will often resolve spontaneously, and patients should be managed with antibiotic therapy and treatment of dysfunctional voiding patterns and constipation. While the use of prophylactic antibiotics is common, it has not been proven by a randomized controlled trial.

The role of surgery is not completely defined, and several controversies exist regarding the value of surgery in the management of this disorder. Elimination of reflux by surgery does not decrease the incidence of mild UTIs, but it may have value in preventing severe pyelonephritis episodes. Since most of the kidney damage occurs during early childhood, surgery must be performed very early in order to be effective.

Since vesicoureteric reflux is a hereditary disorder, screening of at-risk siblings is recommended.

Chapter 7

Nephrolithiasis and Nephrocalcinosis

(CMAJ 2002;166:213)

Introduction: Kidney stone disease is rarely life threatening, but it is a cause of suffering that does result in billions of dollars in health care expenses. Those who suffer one kidney stone have a 60%–80% chance of suffering a recurrence; thus, efforts at prevention of recurrent stones are warranted. Detailed discussion of the urologic management strategies of the stones that do not pass spontaneously is beyond the scope of this book. Most of the emphasis in this chapter is placed on prevention of recurrent stone disease. Whenever possible a recovered stone should be submitted for analysis, as stone composition can guide workup and management. Initial evaluation of patients with recurrent kidney stones should focus on ruling out systemic conditions and medications associated with stone formation.

7.1   Calcium Stone Disease

Cause: Most calcium stones are idiopathic, but a number of systemic conditions can be associated with them, including conditions that lead to hypercalciuria and metabolic acidosis as well as certain medications (see Table 7.1). Anatomic abnormalities of the urinary tract, such as the medullary sponge kidney and congenital megacalyx, can also predispose to stone formation.

Table 7.1 Conditions Associated with Calcium Nephrolithiasis

Hypercalciuria

    Idiopathic
    Secondary to hypercalcemia
        Cancer
        Primary hyperparathyroidism
        Granulomatous diseases
            Sarcoidosis
            Tuberculosis
            Prolonged immobilization
    Drug induced
        Loop diuretics
        Vitamin D intoxication
        Antacids

Drugs Associated with Calcium Stones without Hypercalcemia

    Glucocorticoids
    Non-calcium antacids
    Acetazolamide
    Theophylline

Hyperoxaluria

    Primary hyperoxaluria
    Enteric hyperoxaluria
        Crohn's disease
        Celiac disease
        Pancreatic insufficiency
        Biliary obstruction
        Small intestine bypass (anti-obesity surgery)

Hypocitraturia

    Chronic metabolic acidosis
    Chronic hypokalemia and hypomagnesemia

Epidem: In the United States, calcium stones are by far the most common, comprising nearly 80% of the stones. Kidney stones are more common in the southern and western United States for reasons that may have to do with increased vitamin D production and dehydration in hot climates that lead to lower rates of urine flow. In other areas of the world, such as the Mediterranean basin, uric acid stones are much more common and even constitute the majority of stones in some countries in the Middle East.

Pathophys: Pathophysiology of stone formation is poorly understood. It involves supersaturation of urine and loss of other molecular interactions that prevent stone formation.

Sx: Flank pain, vomiting

Si: Hematuria, flank tenderness

Crs: Stones 4 mm or smaller usually pass spontaneously. Stones larger than 6 mm are unlikely to pass spontaneously and usually require procedures for removal.

Cmplc: Infection, particularly when occurring simultaneously with obstruction and urological complications related to management of stones. Nephrocalcinosis may occur in some patients with recurrent calcium stones.

Lab: There is controversy as to whether patients presenting with the first stone need a workup. Certainly, recurrent stone formers and all children with kidney stones should have a workup, which includes the following labs:

- Stone analysis when possible
- Urinalysis
- Electrolytes
- BUN and Cr
- Ionized calcium and phosphorous
- PTH (particularly if hypercalcemia is present)
- 24-hour urine collection for
  - Volume
  - Sodium
  - Creatinine clearance
  - Calcium

- Uric acid
- Citrate
- Oxalate
- If hyperoxaluria is present, additional workup to rule out all secondary causes of hyperoxaluria (shown in Table 7.1) should be undertaken.

Xray: Kidney stone protocol, noncontrast CT of the abdomen and pelvis, is the best modality for the evaluation of kidney stones.

Rx: After the stones are passed or initial urological procedures have been performed and after systemic conditions such as hyperparathyroidism and other conditions shown in Table 7.1 have been excluded, recurrent calcium stone formers should undergo interventions that will reduce the likelihood of future stone formation:

- Increase water intake to increase daily urine volume to 2.5–3 L. The so-called "stone clinic effect" is the well-documented phenomenon of reduced recurrent stones after attending a "stone clinic." This is believed to be due to the educational value of the advice to increase water intake.
- When hypercalciuria is present, daily urinary calcium excretion should be reduced to 300 mg in men and 250 mg in women. This can be accomplished by treatment with hydrochlorothiazide 25 mg daily. Patients started on hydrochlorothiazide along with a high potassium diet should have their electrolytes measured 1 wk after initiating therapy to screen for hypokalemia and hyponatremia.
- Patients who develop hypokalemia should be treated with potassium citrate instead of potassium chloride, because citrate inhibits stone formation. Excessive administration of citrate can result in metabolic alkalosis, and thus patients who require large doses of potassium citrate for correction of thiazide-induced hypokalemia can be treated with a combination

diuretic that contains amiloride. Triamterene should be avoided as it can cause kidney stones that contain triamterene itself. The unpleasant taste of potassium citrate liquid leads to low compliance with potassium citrate prescription. Urocit-K wax matrix tablets are better tolerated than liquid potassium citrate preparations.

- Hyperoxaluria therapy will vary depending on the cause:
  - Primary hyperoxaluria is a systemic disease that can only be treated with liver transplantation, which will replace the defective enzyme. Short-term urinary alkalinization with citrate can be helpful.
  - Enteric hyperoxaluria should be treated with a low oxalate diet along with optimum management of the underlying gastrointestinal disorder. In some cases, oral administration of calcium carbonate with each meal can bind dietary oxalate and lead to excretion of calcium oxalate in the stool. The goal 24-hour urinary oxalate excretion for these patients is less than 40 mg.
- While there is no evidence that sodium restriction reduces the incidence of recurrent calcium stones, high sodium intake has been associated with increased risk of recurrent calcium stones. Based on this information, most experts recommend reduction in sodium intake that result in 24-hour urinary sodium excretion of less than 3000 mg.
- Hyperuricosuria can lead to formation of uric acid crystals in urine, serving as nuclei that initiate formation of calcium stones. This phenomenon has been observed in approximately 10% of calcium stones. The initial treatment for hyperuricosuria in this setting is a low purine diet. If that does not result in reduction of uric acid excretion, allopurinol at 100–300 mg daily can be used.

7.2 Nephrocalcinosis

(Clin Sci [Lond] 2004;106:549)

Introduction: Nephrocalcinosis is a generalized increase in the calcium content of the kidneys and calcification of renal parenchyma. Nephrocalcinosis usually occurs in the medulla. Cortical nephrocalcinosis may occasionally follow severe cortical injury, such as cortical necrosis.

Cause: Most conditions that cause hypercalciuria can cause nephrocalcinosis. Causes of nephrocalcinosis include:

- Primary hyperparathyroidism
- Renal tubular acidosis
- Bartter's syndrome
- Dent's disease
- Primary or enteric hyperoxaluria
- Oral sodium phosphate colonoscopy preparation (Gastrointest Endosc 2007;65:1102)
- Ethylene glycol ingestion
- Chronic acetazolamide therapy
- Medullary sponge kidney

Epidem: While nephrocalcinosis is a rare cause of renal failure overall, it is relatively common in certain populations such as individuals with enteric hyperoxaluria who have progressive CKD. In certain hereditary conditions such as primary hyperoxaluria and Dent's disease, nephrocalcinosis is the mechanism of kidney disease in the majority of patients.

Pathophys: Intratubular and interstitial calcification are involved in the pathogenesis of this condition. The mechanisms that are responsible for calcification are poorly understood, and it is not clear why some patients develop kidney stones while others may develop extensive medullary calcification with or without stone disease.

Sx: Nephrocalcinosis can be insidious and completely silent. In patients where the condition coexists with stone disease, symptoms related to stone disease will be present.

Crs: The course is highly variable; some patients may develop renal calcification with preservation of renal function while others will have progressive CKD.

Cmplc: Progression to ESRD

Lab: Hypercalciuria and hyperoxaluria will be present in many patients.

Xray: Nephrocalcinosis can be visualized on both plain radiographs and CT. The severity of calcification on imaging studies does not correlate with severity of kidney disease at all.

Rx: Treatment of the underlying condition, such as treatments of bowel disease in enteric hyperoxaluria, parathyroidectiomy for primary hyperparathyroidism, or a liver transplant for primary hyperoxaluria

7.3   Uric Acid Stone Disease

Cause: Uricosuria due to any cause such as:
- High purine or protein intake
- Cell turnover states such as tumor lysis syndrome
- Gout and uricosuric medications

Epidem: Uric acid stones constitute less than 15% of kidney stones in the United States, but they are much more common in some European countries and constitute the majority of stones in some Mediterranean countries.

Pathophys: Uricosuria and acidic urine, along with low urine volume, lead to the formation of uric acid stones.

Sx: Flank pain, vomiting

Si: Hematuria, flank tenderness

Crs: Stones 4 mm or smaller usually pass spontaneously. Stones larger than 6 mm are unlikely to pass spontaneously and usually require procedures for removal. Uric acid stones can dissolve in alkalinized urine.

Cmplc: Infection, particularly when occurring simultaneously with obstruction and urological complications related to management of stones

Lab: Patients with known uric acid stones should have a serum uric acid, a 24-hour urine collection for uric acid, and urinalysis for urine pH.

Xray: Uric acid stones are radiolucent but can be visualized with ultrasound or CT or as filling defects on pyelograms.

Rx: As with calcium stones, increasing the urine volume is the first step in management. Low purine diet should be recommended. Organ meats are particularly high in purines as are beans and some vegetables. Alkalinization of urine with potassium citrate may prevent future stones and lead to dissolution of existing stones. Potassium citrate should be used for urine alkalinization. Patients who cannot tolerate the taste of potassium citrate liquid can be treated with wax matrix Urocit-K tablets. Urine pH can be measured by the patient and therapy adjusted as needed. Patients who develop metabolic alkalosis can be treated with acetazolamide in an attempt to promote excretion of alkaline urine. Patients who cannot achieve the target 24-hour urine uric acid excretion of less than 800 mg can be treated with allopurinol at 100–300 mg daily. Patients allergic to allopurinol can be treated with febuxostat 80–120 mg/d. Febuxostat therapy requires monitoring of liver function tests. (Febuxostat is not yet FDA approved in the US.)

7.4 Struvite Stone Disease

Cause: Struvite stones, also called triple phosphate stones, form in the infected urinary tract.

Epidem: While these stones are relatively rare, they are more common in chronically infected urinary tracts such as in women with chronic UTIs and in patients with chronically infected indwelling devices in their urinary systems.

Pathophys: Urease-producing bacteria alkalinize the urine and produce ammonium. Phosphate then combines with magnesium, calcium, and ammonium to produce struvite. Struvite stones can grow very rapidly in infected urine and can lead to difficult to eradicate infections. Large staghorn calculi are often composed of struvite.

Sx/Si: Patients will have symptoms related to urinary tract infections.

Crs: This disease often follows an aggressive course with rapid stone growth and kidney damage unless infection is rapidly eradicated and/or the stone is removed.

Cmplc: Rapid growth of infected struvite stones can lead to kidney damage and CKD.

Lab: When a patient presents with a large kidney stone, along with a UTI with a urease-producing organism such as proteus, a struvite stone should be suspected.

Xray: CT, ultrasound, and iv urography can be utilized for visualization of these stones.

Rx: Aggressive and prolonged treatment of infection is required when struvite stones are detected. Complete eradication of infection is often impossible when the stone remains in place, and frequent surveillance urine cultures are needed to monitor for recurrence of infection if the stone or stone fragments remain in place. Aggressive urological intervention, such as lithotripsy, or more invasive techniques should be utilized to make the patient stone free and infection free.

7.5 Cystine Stone Disease

Cause: Cystinuria is an inborn error of metabolism that results in the defective renal transport of cystine.

Epidem: 2% of stones in adults and 6%–8% of stones in children

Pathophys: Defective renal tubular transport of cystine, ornithine, lysine, and arginine (COLA) allows large amounts of these amino acids to appear in urine. Cystine can form stones at physiologic pH. Homozygous patients with this disorder can excrete as much as 1000 mg of cystine per day instead of the normal 50 mg. Patients heterozygous for the defective gene excrete less than those with homozygous mutation.

Sx: Flank pain, vomiting

Si: Hematuria, flank tenderness

Crs: Without treatment, multiple stones or staghorn calculi will form by the fourth decade of life.

Cmplc: Complications of stone disease may include obstruction, infection, and CKD.

Lab: 24-hour urine cystine excretion

Xray: Cystine stones are visible on plain radiographs due to high sulfur content.

Rx: Dietary rx is impossible due to the fact that the precursor is an essential amino acid, methionine. High daily urine volumes of at least 4 L are required to dissolve all of the cystine. Cystine is more soluble at a urine pH of more than 7.5, but that is often difficult to accomplish for prolonged periods of time.

Chapter 8

Chronic Kidney Disease

8.1 Approach to a Patient with Chronic Kidney Disease

Introduction: In 2002 the National Kidney Foundation and Kidney Disease Outcome Quality Initiative (KDOQI) issued guidelines to define and classify chronic kidney disease. The impetus for this effort are the poor outcomes in patients with kidney diseases and the high cost of care (Am J Kidney Dis 2002;39:S1).

The criteria for Chronic Kidney Disease (CKD) include:

1. Kidney damage for ≥ 3 months, as defined by structural or functional abnormalities of the kidney, manifest by either:
   - Pathological abnormalities
   - Markers of kidney damage, including abnormalities in the composition of the blood or urine or abnormalities of imaging tests
2. GFR < 60 ml/min/1.73 m^2 for ≥ 3 months

CKD is further stratified into 5 stages based on GFR (see Table 8.1).

It is important to note that the diagnosis of CKD stage 2 should not be made on the basis of GFR alone. There also should be kidney damage present as defined by pathological abnormalities, abnormal imaging, or markers of kidney damage in the blood or urine.

Table 8.1　Stages of Chronic Kidney Disease

Stage	Description	GFR
1	Kidney damage with normal GFR	> 90 ml/min/1.73m^2
2	Kidney damage with mild decrease in GFR	60–89 ml/min/1.73m^2
3	Moderate decrease in GFR	30–59 ml/min/1.73m^2
4	Severe decrease in GFR	15–29 ml/min/1.73m^2
5	Kidney failure or receiving dialysis	< 15 ml/min/1.73m^2

Cause: Diabetes, hypertension, and glomerulonephritis account for most cases of CKD.

Epidem: Approximately 17% of the adult American population has CKD (see Table 8.2; MMWR 2007;56:161). African Americans, Hispanics, and Native Americans are all at increased risk for developing CKD. Risk factors for developing CKD include older age, cardiovascular disease, diabetes, hypertension, and obesity. CKD is also more prevalent in persons with less than a high school education compared to persons with more than a high school education.

Crs: CKD is commonly a progressive disorder. As the kidney function declines, the number of complications increases, as does mortality (see Figure 8.1; N Engl J Med 2004;351:1296).

Table 8.2　Prevalence of CKD in the United States by Stage

Stage	Prevalence
1	5.7 %
2	5.4 %
3	5.4 %
4	0.3 %
5	0.1 %

(MMWR 2007;56:161)

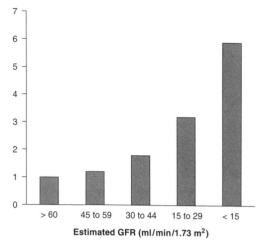

Figure 8.1 Relative Risk of Death in Patients with CKD.

Cmplc:

- Cardiovascular disease
- Hypertension
- Anemia
- Protein energy malnutrition
- Bone disease and disorders of calcium and phosphorous metabolism
- Neuropathy
- Impairments of functioning and well-being

Lab: One of the cornerstone concepts of CKD is staging based on the level of kidney function. The GFR is an excellent measure of kidney function, and declines in GFR are associated with increased risk for complications of CKD and other adverse outcomes. The gold standard for measuring GFR is an inulin clearance. Inulin is a substance that is neither secreted nor reabsorbed by the kidney, so clearance of this substance will equal the GFR. Unfortunately, this test requires an iv infusion and a timed urine collection, which makes it impractical to use for populations with CKD or at risk for CKD. The KDOQI work group evaluated a number of studies to find an estimated GFR that could provide accurate and precise results. The work group concluded that the formula used by the Modification of Diet in Renal Disease (MDRD) study is clinically useful to estimate GFR up to 90 ml/min/1.73 m^2. The formula is based on age, sex, ethnicity, and serum creatinine. The abbreviated form of the formula is:

$$\text{Estimated GFR (ml/min/1.73 m}^2) = 186 \times \\ (\text{serum creatinine(mg/dL)})^{-1.154} \times (\text{age})^{-0.203} \times \\ (0.742 \text{ if female}) \times (1.210 \text{ if African American})$$

This equation can be programmed into handheld calculators, is available for download into PDAs, and is available at www.mdrd.com

Other measures, including the serum creatinine alone and creatinine clearance, were found unreliable. The serum creatinine alone can not provide an accurate estimate for GFR due to the variations of creatinine generation according to age, sex, and other variables. The 24-hour or other timed creatinine clearance is also problematic because of 2 flaws. There is the inherent difficulty of obtaining an accurately timed urine collection. Even if an accurate collection is acquired, the creatinine clearance overestimates the GFR because of proximal renal tubular secretion of creatinine. Thus, the collection of creatinine contains both the filtered and the secreted amounts. This overestimates GFR by 10%-40% in normal subjects but is greater and more unpredictable as the GFR declines. The Cockcroft-Gault equation:

$$\text{Creatinine clearance (ml/min)} = \\ \frac{(140 - \text{age}) \times \text{weight}}{72 \times \text{serum creatine}} \times (0.85 \text{ if female})$$

(weight in kg, serum creatinine in mg/dL)

is a good estimate for creatinine clearance but not for GFR.

24-hour urine testing for creatinine clearance can provide a better estimate of GFR in the following clinical scenarios:

- Vegan diet
- Measurement of residual kidney function for patients on dialysis (see Chapter 9.9)
- Unusual body morphology (eg, amputations)

Patients with CKD should be assessed for abnormal protein excretion in the urine. Acceptable screening tests are a dipstick for protein or albumin, or a spot urine for albumin to creatinine ratio. Any patient with a 1+ or greater dipstick test should undergo quantitative measurement of protein in the urine with a spot urine sample for either albumin to creatinine ratio or protein to creatinine ratio.

Rx: The most important treatment goal for patients with CKD is to prevent progression of kidney disease. Modifiable risk factors for the progression of kidney disease include blood pressure control (see Chapter 10.12), reduction of proteinuria, smoking cessation, and glycemic control for patients with diabetes mellitus. ACEIs and ARBs have a beneficial effect on lowering protein excretion that goes beyond their ability to lower blood pressure. Their use is recommended in patients with diabetic kidney disease with or without hypertension and for patients with hypertension and proteinuria (> 200 mg/g spot protein to creatinine ratio). Other treatment goals are to prevent and treat complications such as:

- Cardiovascular disease (see section 8.2)
- Anemia (see section 8.3)
- Disorders of bone and mineral metabolism (see section 8.4)

If there is difficulty in meeting treatment goals or the estimated GFR is less than 30 ml/min/1.73 m^2, consultation with a specialist is advisable.

8.2 Chronic Kidney Disease and Cardiovascular Disease

KDOQI Clinical Practice Guidelines for Management of Dyslipidemias in Patients with Kidney Disease
(Am J Kidney Dis 2003;41:I)

Cause: Patients with CKD are at increased risk for developing cardiovascular diseases including coronary artery disease, cerebrovascular disease, peripheral vascular disease, and heart failure. Patients with cardiovascular disease risk factors are also at risk for developing CKD.

Epidem: Several epidemiologic studies have demonstrated increased adverse outcomes due to cardiovascular disease in patients with CKD. Data from the Second National Health and Nutrition Examination Survey (NHANES II) demonstrated a higher relative risk of death due to cardiovascular disease (1.68) for participants with estimated GFR < 70 ml/min/1.73 m^2 compared to subjects with estimated GFR > 90 ml/min/1.73 m^2 (J Am Soc Nephrol 2002;13:745). A prospective study of over 1 million patients demonstrated a clear increase in cardiovascular events associated with declining estimated GFR (see Figure 8.2; N Engl J Med 2004;351:1296).

Pathophys: Patients with CKD often have a number of traditional and nontraditional cardiovascular disease risk factors.

Traditional cardiovascular disease risk factors:

- Older age
- Hypertension
- Dyslipidemia
- Diabetes mellitus
- Tobacco use

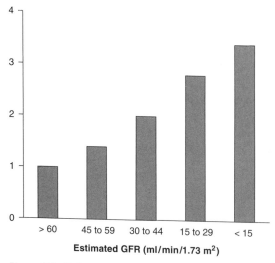

Estimated GFR (ml/min/1.73 m²)

Figure 8.2   Relative Risk of Cardiovascular Events in Patients with CKD.

CKD-related (nontraditional) cardiovascular disease risk factors:

- Decreased GFR
- Proteinuria
- Extracellular fluid volume overload
- Abnormal calcium and phosphorous metabolism
- Anemia
- Malnutrition
- Inflammation
- Renin-angiotensin system activity

Lab: Patients with CKD should have annual screening for risk factors of cardiovascular disease including a complete lipid profile (fasting). Patients with known cardiovascular disease and those at high risk for cardiovascular disease should undergo screening for

CKD with determination of an estimated GFR and screening for proteinuria.

Rx: Patients with CKD should be assessed for modifiable cardiovascular risk factors including cigarette smoking, glucose intolerance, glycemic control, and obesity, at least annually. Patients with CKD should have lower targets for blood pressure and lipoprotein levels. The blood pressure target is 130/80 mm Hg in patients with CKD without proteinuria and 125/75 mm Hg in patients with proteinuria (see Chapter 10.12). An LDL < 100 mg/dL is an appropriate goal in this population. Lifestyle changes and lipid lowering agents may be required to meet goals. Due to the fact that the risk of cardiovascular disease rises as the GFR declines, prevention of progression of CKD is also critical (see section 8.1). Improvements in a number of the modifiable risk factors, including hypertension, glycemic control, and smoking cessation, have the distinction of reducing cardiovascular risk and slowing progression of CKD.

8.3 Anemia Management in End Stage Renal Disease and Chronic Kidney Disease

KDOQI Clinical Practice Guidelines and Clinical Practice Recommendations for Anemia in Chronic Kidney Disease (Am J Kidney Dis 2006;47:S16)

Cause: With the loss of kidney function, the development of anemia is a common outcome for patients with CKD. Erythropoietin deficiency is the most common cause of anemia in patients with CKD. The clinician should not overlook the possible concomitant occurrence of bone marrow disorders, iron deficiency, and chronic inflammation.

Epidem: There are a number of studies that demonstrate a decline in hemoglobin with worsening CKD. The Third and Fourth National Health and Nutrition Examination Surveys (NHANES

III and IV) demonstrated that patients with CKD stages 3 and 4 have much higher rates of anemia than in those with CKD stages 1 and 2 (J Am Soc Nephrol 2002;13:504). Diabetic patients often develop anemia at earlier stages of CKD compared to patients with kidney disease from other causes.

Pathophys: Erythropoietin is the hormone responsible for regulating the production of hemoglobin-containing red blood cells to deliver oxygen to the tissues. It acts on the earliest erythroid precursor cells in the bone marrow, stimulating them to divide and mature into red blood cells. When hemoglobin levels fall, there is a decline in tissue oxygen delivery. The body senses the tissue oxygenation level in cells located in the kidney cortex. These cells increase production of erythropoietin in response to low tissue oxygenation levels.

A number of cofactors are required for this process to be successful. Vitamin B_{12} and folate are necessary for cell division. Adequate iron stores are required for hemoglobin production.

The process can be hindered by the inflammatory cytokines through several mechanisms. They inhibit native kidney erythropoietin production, impair growth of erythrocyte precursors, and interfere with iron metabolism by blocking iron absorption in the gastrointestinal tract and iron release from macrophages.

Sx: Fatigue, lethargy, sexual dysfunction

Si: Pale complexion

Cmplc: Left ventricular hypertrophy is a consequence of untreated anemia due to CKD. There is also increased morbidity and mortality attributable to the lower hemoglobin level.

Lab: Anemia in this group of patients has been defined as a hemoglobin < 13.5 mg/dL for males and < 12 mg/dL for females. KDOQI guidelines advise that patients with CKD be screened annually for anemia. The initial evaluation of a patient with CKD and anemia should include a CBC with differential and platelets along with TSAT and ferritin. Patients with normochromic, normocytic anemia, and normal values for the other cell lines almost always have erythropoietin deficiency if they have CKD stage 3 or higher (estimated GFR < 60 ml/min/1.73 m^2). A serum erythropoietin level can be helpful in patients with earlier stages of CKD.

Rx: One of the main goals of the KDOQI work group has been to improve patient outcomes with guidelines and clinical practice recommendations for patients with CKD and anemia.

Choosing a target hemoglobin level: There is a substantial body of evidence to justify treating patients with anemia and CKD to reach a target hemoglobin of at least 11 mg/dL. Patients on hemodialysis have lower mortality with hemoglobin > 11 mg/dL compared to more anemic patients (J Am Soc Nephrol 1999;10:610). Quality of life measures improve with increased hemoglobin levels. Left ventricular hypertrophy regresses, and hospitalization rates are reduced. In addition, it should be possible to reach a target hemoglobin of 11 mg/dL in the majority of patients.

There have been several studies that have targeted a hemoglobin level higher than 11 mg/dL. The Normalization of Hematocrit (NORMAL) study was done on hemodialysis patients with cardiac disease. The high target group was targeted to reach hematocrit of 42% (hemoglobin 14 mg/dL) compared to a low target group at hematocrit 30% (hemoglobin 10 mg/dL). This study was terminated prior to completion, because the interim statistical analysis demonstrated that it would be extremely unlikely for the high hemoglobin target group to show any benefit, and the high hemoglobin group had a higher incidence of access thrombosis (N Engl J Med 1998;339:584). The Correction of Hemoglobin and Outcomes in Renal Insufficiency (CHOIR) study was done on patients with CKD stages 3 and 4. The high hemoglobin group was targeted to reach a hemoglobin of 13.5 mg/dL, and the low hemoglobin group was targeted to reach 11.3 mg/dL. It also was terminated early when the interim analysis indicated it would be unlikely to show a benefit in the high hemoglobin group. In addition, the overall adverse event rate was higher in the high target group (N Engl J Med 2006;355:2085). The results of these studies indicate that aiming for higher target hemoglobin levels does not provide additional benefit and may even be associated with worse outcomes.

Erythropoietic stimulating agents: ESAs are the mainstay for the treatment of anemia for patients with CKD. The current ESA available to treat anemia due to CKD are recombinant erythropoietin alpha and darbepoetin.

Erythropoietin alpha is usually given at an initial dose of 75 to 150 units/kg weekly. For patients who are on hemodialysis, the weekly dose is usually divided by the number of sessions per week, and the medication is administered iv. For patients who are not on dialysis or who perform peritoneal dialysis, the medication is administered subcutaneously, weekly or biweekly.

Darbepoetin has been designed to be longer acting. It is usually given iv weekly or biweekly to hemodialysis patients and biweekly or monthly via the subcutaneous route to nondialysis or peritoneal dialysis patients. The initial dose of darbepoetin is 0.45 mcg/kg given weekly (0.75 mcg/kg biweekly).

Hemoglobin monitoring should be performed at least monthly for patients on these agents. The dose should be reduced or temporarily discontinued when a rapid rise in hemoglobin is detected. The dose also should be adjusted downward when the hemoglobin is over 12 mg/dL. For patients who do not achieve target within 6 to 8 weeks of therapy, the dose should be adjusted upward. The factors most commonly associated with a failure to achieve target hemoglobin levels are:

- Persistent iron deficiency
- Frequent hospitalizations
- Hospitalization for infection
- Temporary dialysis catheter insertion
- Permanent dialysis catheter insertion

- Hypoalbuminemia
- Elevated C- reactive protein level

Adjuvant iron therapy: The most common reason for a poor response to an ESA is lack of iron. In fact, it is so common that evaluation of iron stores at initiation of ESA therapy and during ESA therapy is clearly indicated. When TSAT levels fall below 20% or ferritin levels are less than 100 ng/ml, iron supplementation will enhance ESA response.

There are several options for iron supplementation. IV iron is the most effective for patients who are on hemodialysis, whereas oral or iv can be useful for nondialysis patients and those on peritoneal dialysis.

The iv iron formulations available are: iron dextran, iron sucrose, and sodium ferric gluconate complex. Oral iron supplements are available in many over-the-counter preparations. The dose to treat iron deficiency in CKO patients should provide approximately 200 mg of elemental iron daily. Each 325 mg tablet of iron sulfate contains 65 mg of elemental iron. Delayed-release formulations, other iron salts, and iron complexes are also available.

To replace deficient iron stores, a dose of 1000 mg of iron is usually sufficient. 100 mg of iron dextran or iron sucrose are given over 10 hemodialysis treatments. Sodium ferric gluconate complex is given in 125 mg doses over 8 sessions. Maintenance of iron stores is achieved with 100 to 125 mg of iv iron monthly. IV iron replacement for patients who are not on dialysis or on peritoneal dialysis can be accomplished with iron sucrose given in 5 doses of 200 mg over a 2-week period.

For patients with ferritin levels greater than 500, iron administration is controversial. If the TSAT is greater than 20%, administration of iron is not indicated. When the TSAT is less than 20% and the patient is still anemic, the clinician needs to decide if ESA responsiveness, hemoglobin level, and the patient's clinical status justify a trial of iron.

8.4 Bone and Mineral Metabolism in End Stage Renal Disease and Chronic Kidney Disease

KDOQI Clinical Practice Guidelines for Bone Metabolism and Disease in Chronic Kidney Disease
(Am J Kidney Dis 2003;42:S1)

Introduction: The manifestations of abnormal bone and mineral metabolism in patients with CKD are:

- Hyperphosphatemia
- Vitamin D deficiency
- Hypocalcemia
- Hyperparathyroidism

Abnormal bone and mineral metabolism begins in the early stages of CKD. Hyperphosphatemia is a consequence of diminished GFR. As kidney function declines, the kidney loses the ability to excrete phosphorous, and phosphorous retention occurs. Vitamin D deficiency develops as the failing kidney is unable to oxidize 25 (OH) vitamin D into the most biologically active form of the vitamin 1,25 (OH) vitamin D (calcitriol). Because one of the functions of vitamin D is to enhance calcium absorption from the diet, hypocalcemia is a consequence of vitamin D deficiency. Chronic hypocalcemia, hyperphosphatemia, and vitamin D deficiency stimulate growth of the parathyroid gland and release of PTH. As time goes on, the hyperplastic tissue releases larger and larger amounts of PTH in response to the stimuli.

Pathophys: The skeletal system and the soft tissues are the target for the manifestations of abnormal bone and mineral metabolism in patients with CKD.

Skeletal system:

- Osteitis fibrosa is a high bone turnover state due to elevated levels of PTH.

- Osteomalacia is due to abnormal mineralization of bones. It is a consequence of inadequate vitamin D levels.
- Adynamic bone disease is a low bone turnover condition, usually caused by over suppression of PTH due to therapy for other forms of renal bone disease.
- Osteoporosis is common in elderly patients with CKD. The etiology is likely multifactorial with hypocalcemia, vitamin D deficiency, and elevated PTH levels all playing a role.

Soft tissues:

- Vascular calcifications can occur in any artery in the body. They cause a significant increase in arterial stiffness. This can be problematic for arteriovenous vascular access creation and other vascular surgical procedures.
- Ocular calcifications can occur on the cornea of the eye and cause corneal irritation.
- Visceral calcifications can occur in the heart, lungs, kidney, and gastrointestinal tract. Complications of cardiac calcifications include CHF, conduction system abnormalities, and valvular calcifications. Pulmonary calcifications can lead to restrictive lung disease and right ventricular hypertrophy.
- Cutaneous calcifications can appear as microscopic deposits within the skin. These can cause pruritis.
- Calcific uremic arteriopathy (calciphylaxis) is a more serious form of cutaneous calcification. Calcification of the dermal arterioles causes local tissue ischemia. The initial manifestations of the condition are localized pain and erythema. It progresses to skin necrosis, which can be extensive. Severe pain and infection often lead to a fatal outcome for this condition.
- Encapsulated solid masses of chalky or paste-like material can also form under the skin. These tumor-like masses are often located near joints.
- Muscle pain is associated with hyperparathyroidism.

- Tendon rupture is associated with hyperparathyroidism.

Epidem: Hyperphosphatemia is associated with increased mortality for patients on dialysis. Patients with serum phosphorous > 6.5 mg/dL have a 1.27 increased relative risk of death compared to patients with phosphorous in the range 2.4 mg/dL to 6.5 mg/dL (Am J Kidney Dis 1998;31:607).

Sx: Bone pain, weakness, pruritis

Si: Bone tenderness; calcium deposits can manifest as conjunctival irritation, palpable masses, skin necrosis

Lab: It is appropriate to begin screening for abnormalities of bone and mineral metabolism for patients who have CKD stage 3 or higher. Annual tests should include:

- Calcium
- Phosphorous
- Intact PTH
- Alkaline phosphatase
- Calculation of the calcium = phosphorous product

For patients on dialysis and undergoing treatment for abnormal bone and mineral metabolism, the testing frequency is increased (see rx for details).

Intact PTH: It is important to obtain a clinically useful measure of the PTH level for patients with CKD. PTH is an 84 amino-acid molecule. The biologically active end is located at the N-terminal. When the PTH is metabolized, there are several inactive fragments created. These fragments are rapidly removed from circulation in patients with normal functioning kidneys but accumulate in patients with CKD. Assays which can not distinguish the fragments from the whole molecule overestimate the level of PTH in patients with kidney failure. The most accurate test to order for patients with CKD is the intact PTH assay.

Alkaline phosphatase: Alkaline phosphatase levels can be elevated in patients with high bone turnover states.

Calcium, phosphorous, and calcium-phosphorous product: The calcium-phosphorous product is calculated by multiplying the calcium level (mg/dL) by the phosphorous level (mg/dL). When the product is over 70 $(mg/dL)^2$, the risk for soft tissue calcifications is increased. Soft tissue calcifications are very rare when the level is below 50 $(mg/dL)^2$.

Xray: The earliest radiologic findings of hyperparathyroidism can be detected on the phalanges. Evidence of subperiosteal bone resorption can be noted as erosion of the distal tuft. Skull and long bone images from patients with long-standing hyperparathyroidism may show a mottled appearance. Vascular calcifications are also often visible on plain films. Technetium-labeled bone scans can demonstrate generalized bone uptake in patients with hyperparathyroidism.

Rx: The KDOQI guidelines for the treatment of abnormal bone and mineral metabolism specify goals for different stages of kidney disease (see Table 8.3).

For patients who are on dialysis (CKD stage 5), the phosphorous goal has been raised in order to allow for more protein to enter the diet. For this population, the goal for PTH is above the normal range in order to avoid over suppression of PTH, which can cause adynamic bone disease.

Table 8.3   Goals for Phosphorous and Intact PTH in Patients with CKD

Stage	Phosphorous goal	Intact PTH goal
CKD stage 3	2.7–4.6 mg/dL	35–70 pg/ml
CKD stage 4	2.7–4.6 mg/dL	70–110 pg/ml
CKD stage 5	3.5–5.5 mg/dL	150–300 pg/ml

Phosphorous control: Dietary phosphorous restriction is the initial approach to managing elevated phosphorous levels. The usual restriction is 800 to 1000 mg daily. See Table 9.12 for a partial list of high phosphorous foods to limit or avoid. Many patients will not reach goal with this therapy alone, so phosphorous binders are often added to the regimen. Phosphorous binders act within the intestinal lumen where they bind to dietary phosphates and block absorption. The most common phosphorous binders available for use are:

- Calcium salts:
  - Calcium carbonate
  - Calcium acetate
- Non-calcium-based binders:
  - Sevelamer hydrochloride
  - Sevelamer carbonate
  - Lanthanum carbonate

Calcium salts: Most patients begin therapy with one of the calcium salts. Several studies have shown these agents to be effective in the majority of patients (Nephrol Dial Transplant 1993;8:341). Some calcium is absorbed when using these agents. This may be beneficial for patients who are hypocalcemic, but in others it can lead to hypercalcemia. For patients who develop hypercalcemia, the calcium in the dialysis bath can be reduced. If this is not effective, the dose of calcium salt should be lowered or another agent should be chosen. For patients who do not reach the phosphorous goal, calcium salts can be combined with other agents for increased effect.

Sevelamer hydrochloride: Sevelamer hydrochloride is an ion exchange resin that binds phosphorous. It can be used alone or in addition to the calcium salts. The serum bicarbonate can fall when switching patients to this agent. This may require a change in bicarbonate concentration for patients on hemodialysis.

Sevelamer carbonate: Sevelamer carbonate works in the same manner as sevelamer hydrochloride. Serum bicarbonate levels improve by approximately 1.3 mcg/L on this binder compared to sevelamer hydrochloride (Clin Nephrol 2007;68:386).

Lanthanum carbonate: This is another noncalcium containing binder. It works in the same manner as calcium salts. It is used alone or in combination with other agents for patients who develop hypercalcemia or who do not reach goal with calcium salts.

    The dialysis process is also effective for lowering phosphorous levels. Patients who perform long nocturnal dialysis sessions often do not require any phosphorous binding agents (Kidney Int 1998;53:1399).

Vitamin D deficiency: It is not uncommon for patients with any stage of CKD to have 25 (OH) vitamin D deficiency. Patients who have this deficiency or suspicion of it can be given ergocalciferol or cholecalciferol supplementation in order to improve bone and mineral metabolism. If they do not show improvement in serum calcium or intact PTH levels they may require calcitriol or a vitamin D analogue.

Hyperparathyroidism:

- Calcitriol and Vitamin D analogues:
  Hyperparathyroidism can persist despite good control of phosphorous and achievement of serum calcium concentration goals. The next step to treat hyperparathyroidism is to add calcitriol or a vitamin D analogue. The agents available for use in addition to calcitriol are paricalcitol, and doxercalciferol. All of the agents are available for iv or oral administration (see Table 8.4).

- The dose of medication can be titrated upward in order to get the intact PTH level to goal. In addition to suppressing PTH secretion, these agents also increase gastrointestinal absorption of calcium and phosphorous. For this reason, it is very important that calcium and phosphorous goals are met

Table 8.4   Dosing of Vitamin D and Vitamin D Analogues in CKD

Medication	Oral Starting Dose	IV Starting Dose
Calcitriol	0.25 mcg daily	1.0 mcg 3 times a week
Paricalcitol	1 mcg daily	2.5 mcg 3 times a week
Doxercalciferol		
CKD stage 3-4	1 mcg daily	
CKD stage 5/dialysis	10 mcg 3 times a week	4 mcg 3 times a week

before initiation of therapy. If there is elevation of calcium, phosphorous, or the calcium-phosphorous product while on therapy, the medication dose should be reduced, or the medication should be discontinued.

Calcimimetics: Calcimimetics increase the sensitivity of the calcium receptor in the parathyroid gland. This causes a decrease in PTH secretion and even reversal of hyperplasia. Cinacalcet is approved for use in patients with ESRD. The indications for initiation of this medication are a PTH level greater than 300 pg/ml and a calcium level greater than 8.4 mg/dL. Unlike the vitamin D analogues, this medication can be started when the phosphorous is above target. Hypocalcemia is the main side effect of the medication. Most patients will also take calcium-containing phosphorous binders. For patients who meet the phosphorous goals, the addition of vitamin D (or vitamin D analogues) can provide additional PTH suppression. The initial dose of cinacalcet is 30 mg daily. The dose is titrated upward to a maximum of 120 mg daily if the PTH level does not reach goal, as long as the serum calcium remains in the normal range. Because this medication can reverse hyperplasia, it often can be titrated to lower doses when used chronically.

Parathyroidectomy: Some patients will develop refractory hyperphosphatemia and refractory hyperparathyroidism despite all of the medical therapies that are available. Often they will also suffer a number of complications of abnormal bone and mineral metabolism, including debilitating soft tissue calcifications, bone pain, and tendon ruptures. When it is clear that all medical therapy has failed, a referral to a surgeon for parathyroidectomy is an option. Since the goal of therapy is to keep the PTH level between 150 and 300 pg/ml, surgical procedures that keep some parathyroid tissue intact are optimal. A subtotal parathyroidectomy where 3 of the 4 glands are removed is one choice. The other is total parathyroidectomy with autotransplantation of some parathyroid tissue in the forearm. The postoperative course of this surgery is notable for profound hypocalcemia, as the bone tissue takes up calcium after the precipitous drop in PTH. This is called the *hungry bone syndrome* and may persist several months. IV administration of calcium is used while the patient is npo. Oral calcium supplementation and vitamin D administration are part of the ongoing management. The dialysis bath calcium level can also be increased.

Laboratory Monitoring: Dialysis patients who are undergoing any therapy for abnormal bone and mineral metabolism should have the calcium and phosphorous levels checked monthly. Intact PTH levels are indicated quarterly. If the patients are initiating therapy with vitamin D, vitamin D analogs, or calcimimetics, the calcium and phosphorous levels can be checked weekly or biweekly and intact PTH levels monthly. Once stable doses of these medications are established the testing frequency can be reduced. Patients who are not on dialysis but are on a phosphorous restricted diet or taking phosphorous binders should have the calcium and phosphorous checked every 3 months.

Chapter 9

End Stage Renal Disease

9.1 Epidemiology of End Stage Renal Disease in the United States

(USRDS Annual Data Report 2006)

Causes: Diabetic patients account for 45% of the new cases of ESRD. More than 90% of these diabetics are type 2. Hypertension, glomerulonephritis, and cystic/hereditary diseases (mostly ADPKD) are the next most common causes of ESRD (see Table 9.1).

Epidem: In 1972 Medicare instituted medical coverage for dialysis and transplantation for patients with ESRD. One of the by-products of this generous program is an extensive database containing facts and figures about the health and demographics of these patients. At the end of 2004, there were over 335,000 people on dialysis in

Table 9.1   Causes of ESRD in the United States by Primary Diagnosis

Primary Diagnosis	Incidence %
Diabetes (overall)	44.9%
Type 1	3.9%
Type 2	41%
Glomerulonephritis	8.2%
Hypertension	24.6%
Cystic/hereditary	3.1%
Urological diseases	4%

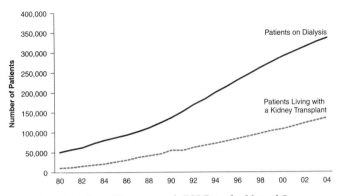

Figure 9.1 Number of Patients with ESRD in the United States.

the United States, and more than 136,000 living with a kidney
transplant. The number of dialysis patients has tripled since 1988
(see Figure 9.1). In 2004, about 102,000 people started dialysis,
about 2000 received a pre-emptive kidney transplant, and about
84,000 patients with ESRD died.

It has been enlightening to examine the trends in incidence
of ESRD over the past several years, and a clear pattern has
evolved. From 1995 to 1999, the incidence growth rate was over
5% per yr, this is dramatically higher than the growth rates from
1999 to 2003, which average just over 1% yearly. Between 2003
and 2004, the incidence rate actually posted a slight decline
(see Figure 9.2). It is difficult to find a definitive reason for the
decline in growth, but hopefully it is due to the improved care
for patients with CKD. Less happily, change in incidence rate of
patients receiving transplants has also declined in this period,
from 5.8% annually for the years 1995 to 1999 to 2.8% annually
for the years 1999 to 2003.

ESRD does not affect all population groups equally. Incidence rates increase with age, and the group with age > 75 has
the highest incidence. Gender and ethnicity also have different

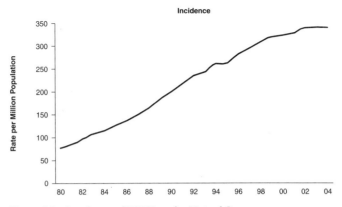

Figure 9.2 Incidence of ESRD in the United States.

rates. Men have nearly twice the rate as women (422 vs. 273 per million). Blacks have 4 times the rate as whites; Native American and Hispanic populations have about double the rate as the white population (see Figure 9.3).

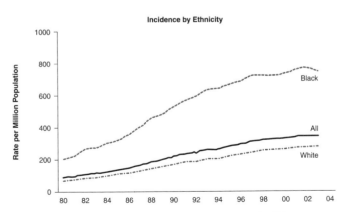

Figure 9.3 Incidence of ESRD in the United States by Ethnicity.

END STAGE RENAL DISEASE

The prevalence rate, which measures the total number of people receiving ESRD therapy in a population, continues to increase (see Figure 9.4). The rate of increase is slowing: from 1995 to 1999, the prevalence rate grew at 5.8% annually, and from 1999 to 2003, it grew at only 2.6%. In 2004 it reached a low of 1.9%. The decline in the growth of the prevalence rate is considerably less than the decline in growth of the incidence rate. The reason that these rates have not declined in tandem is the fact that patients with ESRD are surviving longer. Annual mortality rates have dropped from 289/1000 patients in 1985 to 216/1000 patients in 2004. This represents a 25% decline. Even though these numbers sound encouraging, it is sobering to realize that in 2004, the life expectancy of the average dialysis patient was only 5.6 years, and the life expectancy of the average patient with a kidney transplant was 15.7 years.

The most common reasons for mortality in patients with ESRD are cardiovascular disease and infection. It is also important to note that 22% of the patients who die with ESRD withdraw from dialysis prior to their death.

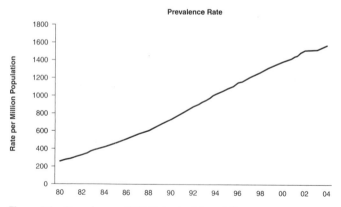

Figure 9.4   Prevalence of ESRD in the United States.

The costs for caring for patients with ESRD in 2004 were a staggering $57,841 per patient that year. The average cost to provide care for a hemodialysis patient was $67,733; peritoneal dialysis patient costs were $48,796 apiece; and it cost $23,840 to provide care for a patient living with a kidney transplant. The cost to provide care for these patients has been increasing annually. The increased prevalence and the increasing yearly costs work together to increase the burden on the Medicare system.

Cmplc:

- Cardiovascular disease (see Chapter 8.2)
- Anemia (see Chapter 8.3)
- Disorders of bone and mineral metabolism (see Chapter 8.4)
- Malnutrition (see section 9.11)

Rx: Initiation of dialysis is a difficult decision for both the patient and the treating physician. For the patient, it means physical changes and challenges, potential economic hardships and a considerable time commitment. For the physician, there is little guidance to optimize the timing of this major therapeutic intervention. There are some clear cut indications for initiation of dialysis in patients with CKD (see Table 9.2).

However, the majority of patients start dialysis without these indications. In any case, since these conditions carry a quantifiable morbidity and mortality, and CKD is often only slowly progressive, it would seem that starting dialysis to avoid these complications would be best. The KDOQI work group advises

Table 9.2 Indications for Initiation of Dialysis

Uremic pericarditis
Fluid overload unresponsive to diuretics
Refractory hyperkalemia
Severe metabolic acidosis
Uremic encephalopathy or neuropathy

that dialysis should be initiated when the GFR is less than 15 ml/min/1.73 m^2 unless none of the following are present: uremic symptoms, fluid overload, and malnutrition (Am J Kidney Dis 2006;48[suppl 1]:S2). This is an opinion-based recommendation. The opinion is partly based on the observation that there is a higher mortality for patients who start dialysis with low serum albumin levels. Trying to determine an optimal GFR at which to begin dialysis has been difficult. Observational studies show that patients who start dialysis with higher GFR have a higher mortality. Part of this observation is due to the fact that these patients also have more comorbidities (Am J Kidney Dis 2005;46:887).

9.2   Hemodialysis Principles and Prescription

Pathophys: The goals of dialysis are to regulate fluid balance and electrolyte composition, while at the same time eliminating a variety of small- and medium-size molecular waste products. Several physical and chemical processes are cleverly deployed to accomplish these tasks. Hemodialysis is performed by pumping blood through a filter consisting of thousands of porous hollow fibers. This filter is often called the *dialyzer*. These fibers are suspended in the dialysate, a customized electrolyte solution that is also pumped through the dialysis filter. Diffusion across a concentration gradient is responsible for much of the electrolyte regulation and waste product elimination. The concentration gradient between the blood and the dialysate is maximized by running the fluids in opposite directions, similar to the counter-current circulation in the loop of Henle (see Figure 9.5). As the blood enters the filter, it will begin the equilibration process with the dialysate that is about to exit the filter, and when the blood is about to return to the patient, it will be dialyzing against a pristine dialysate fluid. Substances can move in either direction across the dialysis membrane. For example, the concentrations of calcium and bicarbonate are often higher in the dialysate than the blood, so a patient will end dialysis with higher levels of these. Levels of potassium, magnesium, and urea are typically reduced. Several factors influence the amount of diffusion that can take place during dialysis. As noted, a concentration gradient is essential. The size of the pores, the total surface area of the capillary tubes, the amount of time the blood and dialysate are in contact, and the permeability of the membrane to the various substances all influence the rate of diffusion.

Ultrafiltration is used to eliminate excess water and sodium during dialysis. This is accomplished by a hydrostatic pressure gradient across the dialysis membrane. Negative pressure is applied to the dialysate, and this pulls an ultrafiltrate consisting of water, sodium, and any other substances that are permeable to the membrane into the dialysate. The main job of ultrafiltration is to remove excess water and sodium, but some waste products and electrolytes are also eliminated. In addition to the pressure gradient, a number of physical properties of the dialyzer membrane influence the rate of ultrafiltrate formation, including the size of the pores, the permeability to water, and the total surface area.

Rx:

See Table 9.3.

- Frequency and length of treatments
  A typical outpatient chronic dialysis prescription has 3 sessions each week lasting for 4 hours. However, the durations often vary from 3 to 5 hours with smaller patients having shorter sessions and larger patients prescribed longer ones. In addition to these conventional prescriptions, there are several other forms available including long duration nocturnal dialysis and short daily dialysis.

  Nocturnal dialysis is performed 3 to 7 times a week, and the sessions are 6 to 8 hours long. This prescription provides

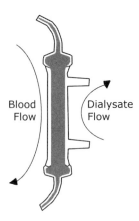

Figure 9.5 Schematic of a Hemodialysis Filter to demonstrate the counter-current flow of blood and dialysate. This maximizes the diffusion gradient for uremic toxins and potassium to diffuse into the dialysate, and bicarbonate and calcium to diffuse into the blood. A negative hydrostatic pressure is applied across the semipermeable membrane, which facilitates the movement of water, sodium, and other small molecules from the blood into the dialysate.

Table 9.3 Components of the Hemodialysis Prescription

Frequency of treatments
Length of treatment
Dialyzer: Size and membrane type
Blood flow rate
Dialysis flow rate
Dialysis bath potassium concentration
Dialysis bath calcium concentration
Dialysis bath bicarbonate concentration
Anticoagulation during dialysis (usually heparin based)
Ultrafiltration goal or dry weight

twice as much dialysis as thrice weekly treatments. There are several clinical benefits to this schedule including better control of blood pressure, anemia, and bone and mineral metabolism (Kidney Int 2005;67:1500). Despite these excellent outcomes, only a small fraction of patients are on this program. There are patient and institutional barriers to further acceptance of this program. Patient barriers include a longer time commitment and the training required to provide self care in the home. Institutional barriers include current Medicare reimbursement policies, which make it difficult to obtain reimbursement for more than 3 dialysis sessions per week.

Daily short dialysis is performed in the home setting, and the sessions are 1.5 to 2 hours in duration 6 times weekly. Clinical outcomes of daily short dialysis compare well to conventional schedule (Nephrol Dial Transplant 2005;20:285). The patients who perform this have more freedom to schedule their treatments and more control of their care.

- Dialyzer

Dialysis filters can be ordered based on the size of pores (high flux/large pore or low flux/smaller pore), membrane material (synthetic vs cellulose based), and surface area. Current KDOQI recommendations are to use high-flux dialysis filters. The Hemodialysis (HEMO) study demonstrated improved clinical outcomes in patients dialyzed with high-flux dialysis filters compared to low flux dialysis filters (N Engl J Med 2002;347:2010). The high-flux dialyzer is permeable to beta-2 microglobulin, which is responsible for dialysis-related amyloidosis. That substance and other mid-sized waste products may be responsible for some of the morbidity and mortality of uremia. Potential pitfalls of high-flux dialysis are the backflow of substances from the dialysate into the patient, including potentially harmful compounds such as endotoxin fragments (Semin Dial 2004;17:489) and more rapid movement of ultrafiltrate across the membrane. Thus, the generation of very pure dialysate and exact measurement of the ultrafiltration volume are important components in delivering safe high-flux dialysis.

Cellulose-based and synthetic membranes are available in high-flux formulations, but the optimal choice of membrane material remains controversial. Cellulose-based membranes can activate complement, which could lead to an inflammatory state. The synthetic membranes do not do this and are called *biocompatible*. Despite this difference, most studies have not shown a morbidity or mortality difference attributable to membrane material (Cochrane Database Syst Rev 2005;CD003234).

The dialyzer surface area is usually chosen based on the patient's size. It is not uncommon to increase the dialyzer size in order to increase the amount of dialysis a patient receives. A larger dialyzer requires more extracorporeal blood to be in the dialysis circuit and that may cause hypotension in some patients.

- Blood and dialysate flow rates
  The rate of blood flow through the dialyzer is limited by physical trauma that could occur when pumping at high rates of speed. The highest safe rate with the current tubing, dialyzers, and blood pumps is about 400 ml/min. The dialysate rate is usually chosen to be twice the blood flow rate. More than this ratio does not provide a significant increase in the concentration gradient for diffusion to occur.

- Dialysis bath
  The dialysis bath is created by mixing concentrated electrolyte solution with very pure water. The sodium concentration of the final mixture ranges from 135 to 145 mEq/L. The most common potassium concentration ordered is 2.0 mEq/L. For patients with hyperkalemia, the potassium value can be lowered to 1.0 mEq/L; however, a potassium-free dialysate is risky and associated with increased rate of death (Kidney Int 2001;60:350). The calcium concentration usually varies

from 2.0 to 3.5 mEq/L. The normal ionized calcium concentration in the blood is approximately 2.5 mEq/L, so patients who are hypercalcemic are dialyzed against the low-calcium bath, and patients who are hypocalcemic are dialyzed against the higher calcium baths. Use of a calcium-free bath is not advised because it can lead to cardiac instability. The standard bicarbonate concentration is 35 mEq/L; this provides an infusion of bicarbonate to dialysis patients who usually have a mild metabolic acidosis.

A 4-hour dialysis session requires the creation of nearly 200 L of water (see Figure 9.6). Since the patient is directly exposed to this, the AAMI has set very high quality standards for the biological and chemical purity of water. In order to be in compliance with the Medicare Conditions for Coverage, a dialysis provider must meet or exceed these standards. Several additives to municipal water supplies can have detrimental health effects on dialysis patients. Alum, which helps remove particulate matter, contains aluminum. Long-term exposure to aluminum can lead to dementia. Acute fluoride exposure can cause cardiac arrest (Ann Intern Med 1994;121:339). Exposure to chloramines, a common sanitizing agent, causes hemolytic anemia (Rev Saude Publica 2001;35:481). AAMI standards dictate that the water is completely analyzed for chemical contaminants several times a year. It must be tested daily for chloramines. Biological purity is assured by regular bacterial culture of the water system and regular assays for endotoxins.

- Anticoagulation
  The process of circulating blood through the dialysis filter and back to the patient exposes the blood to numerous thrombogenic stimuli. In order to prevent extracorporeal thrombosis and the resulting blood loss, almost all patients are anticoagulated during the dialysis session. Unfractionated heparin is the most commonly employed agent. The usual dosing is to give a bolus based on the patient's weight (approximately 50 units/

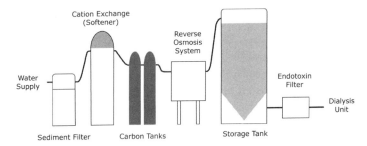

Figure 9.6 A Typical Hemodialysis Water Treatment System. The cation exchanger (softener) removes calcium and magnesium, which can damage the membranes of the reverse osmosis component. Carbon tanks remove chlorine and chloramines and other dissolved organic substances. The reverse osmosis unit removes all other impurities to provide chemically and microbiologically pure water to the dialysis unit.

kg) and then run a continuous infusion of 500 to 1000 units/hr until 30 minutes prior to the end of the treatment. The dose of the bolus and the infusion is adjusted empirically based on any clotting episodes or prolonged bleeding from dialysis needle puncture sites. Measurement of the activated clotting time or PTT can also be used to establish anticoagulation. In order to meet Clinical Laboratory Improvement Amendments (CLIA) standards, these measurements must be made by a certified laboratory. This is rarely done in outpatient settings.

A rare but troublesome complication of heparin anticoagulation is the development of heparin-induced thrombocytopenia. Options for patients like this include anticoagulation using argatroban or heparin-free dialysis. Argatroban can be given as a single dose at the onset of the treatment (Kidney Int 2004;66:2446). Heparin-free dialysis is performed by flushing the dialysis circuit every half hour with normal saline. Results of heparin free dialysis are surprisingly successful, as over 80% of treatments are without significant thrombotic events (Hemodial Int 2005;9:393).

Low molecular heparin is another agent that can be used for anticoagulation; enoxaparin can be given as a single initial dose of 40 mg (J Am Soc Nephrol 2004;15:3192).

- Ultrafiltration goal/dry weight

The amount of fluid to remove at a dialysis session is usually calculated as the amount of weight a patient has gained in the intradialytic interval. This is based on the concept that at the end of dialysis a patient will be at his or her dry weight. Over the short term, the dry weight is unlikely to change; however, over the longer term, a patient may gain or lose some dry weight, and an adjustment is required. Patients who have symptoms of hypovolemia at the end of dialysis may need their dry weights adjusted higher, and patients who still have edema or hypertension at the end of dialysis may need their dry weights reduced. The rate of fluid removal is also important. Since the ultrafiltrate is removed directly from the vascular space, high rates of ultrafiltration often cause symptomatic hypotension even if the extravascular compartment still has signs of fluid overload. Patients with high fluid goals may need longer and more frequent dialysis sessions in order to reach their dry weight.

9.3 Hemodialysis Access

Clinical Practice Guidelines for Vascular Access
(Am J Kidney Dis 2006;48[suppl 1]:S248; J Nephrol 2001;14:532)

Introduction: Vascular access is an essential yet vexing prerequisite for the performance of chronic hemodialysis. In 2003 nearly 1.5 million vascular access procedures were performed on hemodialysis patients (USRDS 2006 Annual Data Report). This averages over 4 procedures for each patient. There are 3 choices of vascular access that account for nearly 100% of the access in use today: arteriovenous fistula (AVF), arteriovenous graft (AVG), and double lumen catheter. The AVF is the preferred access because patency rates are 3 to 4 years compared to 2 years for AVGs and only 1 year for catheters. Infection rates for AVFs are also lower than for other forms of access. In fact, patients dialyzed with AVFs have better long-term morbidity and mortality compared to patients dialyzed with AVGs or catheters (Nephrol Dial Transplant 1997;12:657).

Pathophys:

- AVF
  To create an AVF the surgeon connects the vein to an artery in an end (of vein) to side (of artery) anastomosis. This allows for a dramatic increase in the blood flowing through the vein while preserving downstream flow of blood through the artery. Once the anastomosis is complete, the high rate of blood flow through the vein will stimulate an increase in the diameter of the vein and a thickening of the wall of the vessel. The maturation process typically takes 2 months. Not surprisingly, veins with a minimum diameter of 3.5 mm and arteries with a minimum diameter of 2.5 mm have higher rates of success (Eur J Vasc Endovasc Surg 1996;12:207). The first choice for the location of the AVF is at the wrist (see Figure 9.7). If an AVF can be established here, it is likely to have a very long patency period (Nephrol Dial Transplant 2004;19:1231). Many patients do not have adequate vessels in the wrist, including diabetics and the elderly (Am J Kidney Dis 2002;39:1218). For these patients, the second choice is an AVF at the elbow. There are 2 choices for outflow vein for these fistulas. The cephalic vein or the deeper basilic vein can be used. The basilic vein is less often damaged from repeated venipuncture, but the procedure to connect it is more complicated. It usually needs to be brought closer to the surface and transposed from

the medial side of the arm to the palmar side to allow for easier cannulation.

It is important to refer the patient to a surgeon for creation of the AVF well before the patient is on dialysis. There is decreased mortality and morbidity in patients who start dialysis with a fistula compared to other forms of vascular access (Am J Kidney Dis 2003;42:1013). Procedures to create an AVF have a 25% failure rate, and it takes 2 months or more for a fistula to mature. Current KDOQI recommendations are to begin this process when the patient reaches CKD stage 4 (estimated GFR 15-25 ml/min/1.73 m^2.

- AVG

An AVG is created by placing a synthetic vein graft between the artery and vein. The most common material used for the creation of an AVG is polytetrafluoroethylene (PTFE). A variety of other materials have been used, and to date there is no advantage to any particular material (Semin Vasc Surg 2004;17:19). AVGs are usually located in the upper extremity. Possible configurations include: a straight graft from the

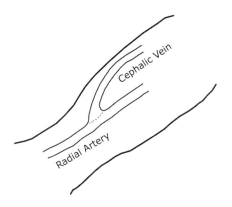

Figure 9.7 AVF at the Wrist.

wrist to elbow, a loop at the elbow, or a straight graft from the elbow to upper bicep area. Similar to the AVF, initial success depends on the size of the available arteries and veins. A loop or straight graft below the elbow is preferred to more proximal placement in order to preserve as many potential sites as possible. For patients who have exhausted upper extremity sites, a loop graft can be placed in the thigh with similar patency results to upper extremity AVGs (J Am Soc Nephrol 2003;14:2942). An AVGs typically only takes a few weeks to mature in order to be ready for cannulation.

A secondary AVF can be created in a patient with a pre-existing AVG. After several months or even years, the outflow vein from the AVG often increases in diameter and wall thickness due to high blood flow. A secondary AVF is created by connecting this mature outflow vein directly to an artery. It often can be used for dialysis immediately, without the need for a dialysis catheter (Semin Dial 2005;18:420). The KDOQI recommendations are to consider this operation at each instance of AVG malfunction; however, even this may result in some missed opportunities, so it is probably better to proactively examine all patients with AVGs for the existence of a suitable venous channel for conversion. This is easily done at the bedside.

- Dialysis catheter
  Chronic hemodialysis can be performed using a large bore central venous catheter as well. The catheter is designed with 2 lumens. The inflow lumen (somewhat misleadingly labeled the arterial lumen) has multiple holes along its proximal aspect. The outflow (venous) lumen channels the blood out of more distally located holes and out the distal end of the catheter. This design reduces the possibility of blood recirculation during dialysis. The optimal location for the catheter is the right internal jugular vein. The subclavian veins are a poor choice due to possibility of developing subclavian stenosis. Catheter

placement using ultrasound guidance has better success and less complications (Nephrol Dial Transplant 1997;12:1234). The use of venography to identify any venous anatomical anomalies may also reduce complications (Nephrol Dial Transplant 2004;19:1542). The catheter tip position should be confirmed by Xray (or fluoroscopy) to be located in the right atrium. Most catheters used for long-term dialysis are tunneled through the skin to exit on the anterior chest. They also have a cuff, which stimulates tissue growth subcutaneously that secures the catheter in place and seals the skin from the intravascular space. Noncuffed catheters can be used for short-term dialysis (approximately 1 week).

Epidem: In the United States, 19% of patients are dialyzed with a catheter, 36% with an AVF, and 55% with an AVG (USRDS Annual Data Report 2006). Fistula rates in the United States demonstrate a distinct geographic variability where the northeastern states and northwestern states have rates higher than the southeastern states. The rates in the United States as a whole do not compare favorably with many other countries. This has not been able to be explained by any patient characteristics. It seems that local physician practice patterns are responsible (Kidney Int 2003;64:681). Because of this, the KDOQI and Healthy People 2010 began the Fistula First initiative in 2004. The Fistula First program has set a goal of 66% AVF usage for the nation by 2009. In order to achieve this goal, this program distributes educational materials for patients and physicians about the positive impact on life expectancy with AVFs and provide feedback to local dialysis units about access rates. This program is having an excellent impact on increased AVF rates over the whole country, with a 30% increase in fistula use for the entire United States from December 2002 to June 2007. Even higher rates of increase have been noted in locations of low AVF prevalence (www.fistulafirst. org).

Unfortunately, the number of patients who start dialysis with a catheter has trended upward since 1988 (USRDS 2006 Annual Data Report:115). The increase in the population of elderly and diabetic patients correlates with the increase in catheter usage. The KDOQI work group has set a goal to reduce the dialysis catheter rate to 10%.

Cmplc: See sections 9.5 and 9.6.

Thrombosis is the cause of 80% of AVG and AVF failure. Other serious complications include infections and steal syndrome. An AVF can form aneurysmal dilation over time. AVGs are prone to pseudo-aneurysms, which develop when the graft material breaks down after repeated cannulation. Dialysis catheter infection and dialysis catheter malfunction causing low flow are all too frequent occurrences. Catheter insertion complications include pneumothorax, arterial puncture, and blood loss. Central vein stenosis is a potential consequence of an indwelling catheter.

9.4   Hemodialysis Adequacy

Clinical Practice Guidelines for Hemodialysis Adequacy, Update 2006 (Am J Kidney Dis 2006;48[suppl 1]:S2)

Pathophys: Adequate dialysis is defined as the dose of dialysis required to optimize the patient's survival and health. There are a number of studies that show that inadequate dialysis is associated with higher rates of death and hospitalization.

Lab: The simplest way to measure the adequacy of dialysis is to compare the BUN at the beginning of dialysis to the BUN at the end of the treatment. The urea reduction ratio (URR) is calculated from these 2 measurements with the following equation:

$$\text{URR} = \left[1 - \left(\frac{\text{Postdialysis BUN}}{\text{Predialysis BUN}} \right) \right] \times 100\%$$

Using these terms, a URR of 70% would indicate that 70% of the BUN was removed during a dialysis session. This statistic has been very useful for studying the effect of the dose of dialysis on large populations of dialysis patients. These studies have revealed that a URR < 65% is associated with increased morbidity and mortality.

Although the URR is a good measure of dialysis dose for population-based studies, it is not a very accurate measurement of the amount of dialysis a patient receives. The formula does not take into account the urea removed with the ultrafiltration volume, the amount of urea removed from the residual function of the native kidneys, or the amount of urea generated during the time of a dialysis treatment. In order to account for all these variables, urea kinetic modeling has been developed as another way to measure the dose of dialysis. When using urea kinetic modeling to measure dialysis, the dose of dialysis is measured as the $K_{urea}T_d/V_{urea}$ (Kt/V); where T_d is the length of time of the dialysis session, V_{urea} is the volume of distribution of urea, and K_{urea} is the dialyzer urea clearance. There are a number of formulae and even computer simulations that can calculate the Kt/V. The KDOQI work group published guidelines in 2006 that advise the use of the following formula to calculate the Kt/V:

$$Kt/V = -\ln(R - 0.008 \times t) + (4 - 3.5 \times R) \times \frac{\Delta BW}{BW}$$

where $R = \dfrac{\text{Postdialysis BUN}}{\text{Predialysis BUN}}$, t = time in hours and BW is body weight measured in kg.

In terms of Kt/V, a value of 1.2 is considered to provide adequate hemodialysis. A number of clinical studies have been done using Kt/V, which shows that values less than 1.2 are associated with increases in morbidity and mortality. In addition, the HEMO study did not show that increasing Kt/V to 1.5 offered any increased benefit to most dialysis patients (J Am Soc Nephrol 2003;14:1863).

Rx: Current KDOQI recommendations are to measure the dose of dialysis monthly. Kt/V is the preferred measurement. The goal is to provide a Kt/V of 1.4. The goal is set higher than the minimum because any technical problems (or scheduling ones) often result in delivering a smaller dose of dialysis to the patient than the prescribed dose. If the Kt/V is below target, steps to increase it should be initiated. These include increasing the time (t) on dialysis. The K_{urea} can also be increased by increasing the size of the dialyzer, increasing the blood and dialysate flow through the dialyzer, or improving the dialysis access to either provide better flow or less access recirculation.

Access Recirculation

Clinical Practice Guidelines for Hemodialysis Adequacy, Update 2006 (Am J Kidney Dis 2006;48[suppl 1]:S2)

Cause: Access recirculation is due to the dilution of blood entering the dialysis circuit with blood that has been already dialyzed.

Pathophys: When a stenosis is present in the venous end of the blood dialysis access, the obstruction impedes blood leaving the dialysis circuit, and will flow in a retrograde manner back into the arterial supply. Access recirculation also can be due to poor arterial inflow. When the arterial supply is low, the dialysis machine's arterial pump will actually siphon blood from the venous outflow to make up for the arterial shortage. Incorrect placement of needles can also increase access recirculation. When the arterial and venous needles are too closely spaced, there can be mixing of the blood supplies. If the needles are placed in the reverse sequence, eg, the arterial needle is placed more proximal to the venous needle, venous blood will enter the circuit. This can easily happen when the dialysis access is in a loop, and the nurse or technician does not know which direction the blood flows through the loop. Dialysis catheters are designed with the arterial openings located more proximally (on the catheter) compared to the venous return, which includes the distal end. Often a poorly performing catheter will be connected in a reversed manner in order to improve blood flow. This can increase recirculation values to as high as 15% (Am J Kidney Dis 2005;45:883).

Compl: When access recirculation values are elevated, the effectiveness of the dialysis process is decreased. Inadequate dialysis and hyperkalemia are potential adverse outcomes. Because it is often associated with a stenosis in an arteriovenous access, access thrombosis is a likely consequence if left untreated.

Lab: Access recirculation can be calculated by measuring the BUN entering the dialysis circuit (BUN arterial), the BUN leaving the circuit (BUN venous), and the peripheral BUN (BUN peripheral).

The percent recirculation is calculated:

$$\% \text{ recirculation} = \left(\frac{\text{BUN peripheral} - \text{BUN arterial}}{\text{BUN peripheral} - \text{BUN venous}} \right) \times 100$$

When there is no recirculation, the BUN peripheral and the BUN arterial are equal, and the numerator of the equation is zero. As the recirculation increases, the arterial blood will be diluted by the already dialyzed venous blood, which will decrease the arterial BUN value. The samples for the BUN arterial and BUN venous can be obtained from the appropriate ports on the dialysis tubing. The peripheral BUN can be obtained in the contralateral arm or from the arterial port of the dialysis tubing after decreasing the blood flow through the system to 50 ml/min or less. This latter method essentially eliminates any possibility of venous blood diluting the arterial supply. Access recirculation can also be measured by dilution techniques, similar to the ones used to noninvasively measure access flow.

END STAGE RENAL DISEASE

Rx: Access recirculation values greater than 10% should prompt referral for imaging of the access and repair if needed. Other methods to reduce recirculation include replacement of a poorly performing dialysis catheter and appropriate placement of needles in the access. For loop-shaped dialysis access, it is important for the person who places the needles to be familiar with the operative note describing the flow direction.

9.5 Complications of Arteriovenous Fistulas and Arteriovenous Grafts

Thrombosis and Stenosis in AVF and AVG

Clinical Practice Guidelines for Vascular Access (Am J Kidney Dis 2006;48[suppl 1]:S248)

Causes: The root causes of access thrombosis are factors that decrease blood flow and hypercoagulable states.

- Low flow:
  - Stenosis of the venous end of the access accounts for 85% of thrombotic episodes
  - Arterial inflow stenosis
  - External compression of the access
  - Hypotension
- Hypercoagulable states
  - Antiphospholipid antibody syndrome (including Lupus anticoagulant)
  - Factor V Leiden mutations
  - Protein C deficiency
  - Protein S deficiency
  - Antithrombin III deficiency
  - Heparin-induced thrombocytopenia
  - Rapid rise in hct associated with erythropoiesis

Table 9.4   KDOQI Thrombosis and Patency Goals for AVF and AVG

	Goal
Annual AVG thrombosis rate	< 0.5 episodes/patient
AVG patency	> 2 years
Annual AVF thrombosis rate	< 0.25 episodes/patient
AVF patency	> 3.0 years

Epidem: The rate of access thrombosis is approximately 0.8 episodes/ patient/year at risk. Single or repeated episodes of thrombosis account for most access failure. The expected patency of an AVG is only 2 years. The expected patency of an AVF is 3 years. Wrist AVFs have the longest patency at 5 years. KDOQI, goals for thrombosis and patency have been set: see Table 9.4.

Pathophys: The chain of events that ends in thrombosis usually starts with a stenosis.

An area of stenosis is histologically characterized by vascular endothelial cell proliferation and inflammatory cell infiltration. The stenosis is thrombogenic in nature due to the increase in inflammatory mediators and platelet aggregation factors. Although stenosis can occur anywhere in an arterio-venous access, there are a number of predisposing factors for cell proliferation in the venous limb of an AVG. Vascular wall injury, turbulent blood flow, shear stress, and elastic mismatch of the artificial material compared to the native vein are all present.

Si: Clinical assessment of the patient with notation of swollen arm, difficult cannulation, or prolonged bleeding at the end of dialysis can signal imminent access failure. These are good indications to perform a fistulogram.

Lab: Workup for hypercoagulable states should be considered when there are recurrent episodes of vascular access thrombosis without anatomic cause. Typical testing would include screening for lupus anticoagulant, factor V Leiden mutations, anticardiolipin antibodies, and deficiencies of protein C, protein S, and ATIII. Any patient with the combination of thrombocytopenia and vascular access thrombosis should also be evaluated for heparin-induced antiplatelet antibodies.

Xray: A key to preventing thrombosis is the detection of vascular access stenosis (Am J Kidney Dis 1998;32:302). A fall in access blood flow and low access blood flow are the most sensitive predictors of stenosis. There are a number of ways to measure blood flow in the access. Thermodilution techniques can be used during the dialysis treatment. Duplex and Doppler ultrasounds are also accurate. Regular determination of flow should be performed. When a fall in blood flow of 20% from the baseline or a rate below 600 ml/min for AVG and below 450 ml/min for AVF is detected , the access should be evaluated by fistulogram for stenosis.

A number of other factors also predict thrombosis. An increase in the venous pressure readings during dialysis can indicate stenosis of the venous end of the access. Increased access recirculation is usually associated with critical access stenosis. Dialysis accesses with these findings should be evaluated by fistulogram.

Rx: Treatment options for a thrombosed fistula or graft include surgical thrombectomy, percutaneous techniques, and systemic thrombolysis. Since an underlying stenosis is responsible for so many of these thrombotic episodes, repair of the stenosis is critical to the long-term success of any procedure.

Surgical thrombectomy has a very high success rate for restoring access flow. Its disadvantages are that it exposes the patient to the risks of anesthesia, and unless the underlying stenosis is not repaired, a recurrent thrombosis is inevitable. If a fistulogram and surgical revision can not be performed at the same setting, they should be scheduled to be done as soon as possible.

Percutaneous techniques to remove the clot include mechanical thrombectomy and local administration of thrombolytic agents. During the same session, a fistulogram can be performed, and any stenotic lesions can undergo angioplasty. Percutaneous interventions should be performed in a timely fashion as clots more than 48 hours old have a 2-fold higher rate of technical failure (Kidney Int 2000;57:1169).

Systemic thrombolysis is a rarely used option. Only a limited number of dialysis patients are eligible due to the inherent risks. In addition, this procedure should be accompanied by a fistulogram and plans to repair any stenotic lesion.

The treatment of stenosis is based on the fistulogram findings. Any stenosis greater than 50% is potentially thrombogenic and should be treated. Treatment options include angioplasty or surgical revision. Success rates are similar with the 2 procedures. Each institution should decide on the optimal strategy with the resources that are available. Once the procedure has been completed, measurement of the access flow should be made to get a new baseline.

Warfarin has been used to reduce the number of episodes of vascular access thrombosis in patients with hypercoagulable states. Systemic anticoagulation has not been successful in the dialysis population as a whole to reduce access thrombosis. Warfarin, aspirin, dipyridamole, and even combinations of these have been trialed without success (Am J Kidney Dis 2002;40:1255).

Infections in AVF and AVG

Clinical Practice Guidelines for Vascular Access (Am J Kidney Dis 2006;48[suppl 1]:S248)

Causes:

- Postoperative infection
- Pseudoaneurysm
- Infected hematoma
- Local skin infection
- Endogenous infection from other site (eg, endocarditis)

Epidem: Infection accounts for approximately 20% of arteriovenous vascular access loss.

Patients with AVGs have higher infectious-related death rate than patients with AVFs (J Am Soc Nephrol 2004;15:477).

Pathophys: Typically, these infections are from skin-based flora-like staphylococci and streptococci, but because patients with ESRD have compromised immune systems, Gram negative organisms and enterococci are not infrequent.

Si: Local signs of inflammation: redness, swelling, pain

Systemic signs of infection: fever

An exposed graft or purulent drainage from a sinus tract is a sure sign of an infected AVG.

Cmplc: An occult infection of a nonfunctioning AVG can be responsible for a poor response to erythropoietin and other signs of chronic inflammation, including hypoalbuminemia.

An intense local inflammatory response can occur following AVG insertion. This can be a challenge to differentiate from a postoperative infection. Edema is common in both settings. The local reaction is characterized by redness along the entire length of the AVG. A postoperative infection is usually located near the surgical incisions, can have associated purulence, more far-reaching cellulitic signs, and systemic signs of infection including fever, elevated wbc, and positive blood cultures. It is important to examine and re-examine the patient with a new AVG in the early postoperative phases, as the intense local reaction will also subside without antibiotic treatment over the course of a few days.

Systemic bacteremia is a consequence of an infected graft with potential hematogenous spread to other tissues, including heart valves and bones.

Lab: CBCD, blood cultures, wound cultures

Xray: Indium-labeled wbc scan can detect occult infection of thrombosed AVG.

Rx: An infected AVF should be treated with 6 weeks of antibiotic therapy. Initial therapy should include coverage for *Staphylococcus aureus*. If an AVG has a localized area of infection, antibiotics and partial resection of the graft is the appropriate initial treatment. This will fail approximately 25% of the time but can avoid placement of a dialysis catheter. If this treatment fails or if there is extensive infection of the graft, total resection of the graft should be undertaken (J Vasc Surg 2004;39:73). Patients with sepsis should also undergo total graft removal. Initial antibiotic choice for an infected AVG should include staphylococcal, streptococcal, and Gram-negative coverage. Continued therapy should be based on culture results.

Aneurysms

Clinical Practice Guidelines for Vascular Access (Am J Kidney Dis 2006;48[suppl 1]:S248)

Cause: Aneurysms develop in AVFs that have undergone repeated cannulation in a relatively limited area. If an aneurysm develops in an area that is not being cannulated, there is likely a stenosis in the outflow vein just proximal to the aneurysm. AVGs develop pseudoaneurysms due to breakdown of the graft material after repeated cannulation.

Cmplc:

- Skin breakdown of the overlying skin
- Rupture
- Infection
- Limited number of cannulation sites

Rx: Aneurysms and pseudoaneurysms should not undergo cannulation. If a stenosis is suspected as the cause of the aneurysm, partial resection of the aneurysm wall and surgical revision of the stenosis is the first treatment choice. Angioplasty is a second option. Other indications for partial resection or surgical revision include: rapid change in size, compromise of the overlying skin, and limitation of the number of cannulation sites.

Vascular Steal Syndrome

Cause: The arteriovenous vascular access diverts a significant portion of the blood that would normally go to the extremity distal to the access. In addition, flow through the palmar arch can provide retrograde flow into a forearm vascular access compromising the blood supply to the digits. Vascular steal syndrome occurs when there are signs and symptoms of ischemia in the extremity. It is almost always seen in conjunction with peripheral vascular disease. Some cases are associated with very high rates of blood flow through the access.

Epidem: Several studies show that symptomatic steal syndrome develops in about 10% of patients with AVFs or AVGs. It can develop within 24 hours of the surgical procedure—especially in the case of AVG creation. It can take several months to develop after AVF creation (Nephrol Dial Transplant 2003;18:2387).

Si: See Table 9.5.

Crs: Mild symptoms (stage 1) are quite common after initial access creation; often collateral vessels will develop, and symptoms will resolve.

Cmplc: Nonhealing ulcers, ischemic nerve damage

Xray: Duplex ultrasound, fistulogram

Table 9.5 Stages of Vascular Steal Syndrome Associated with AVF or AVG (Am J Kidney Dis 2006;48 Suppl 1:S248)

Stage 1	Pale, blue or cold hand without pain
Stage 2	Pain during exercise or during hemodialysis
Stage 3	Pain at rest
Stage 4	Any one or a combination of ulcers, necrosis and gangrene

Rx: Treatment should be based on the results of the vascular studies (Am J Kidney Dis 2006;48:88). For patients with peripheral vascular disease, noninvasive options include angioplasty of any proximal stenosis in the extremity. The most successful surgical procedure is distal revascularization with interval ligation (DRIL) (Semin Vasc Surg 2004;17:45). In this operation, the stenotic lesion undergoes a bypass, and the artery distal to the arteriovenous anastomosis is ligated. The second part of the procedure prevents any retrograde flow into the vascular access. For cases where there is excessive blood flow through the access, a surgical banding procedure is recommended. Ligation of the outflow vein of the access may be necessary when the viability of the limb is at risk.

9.6   Dialysis Catheter Complications

Dialysis Catheter Infection

(Semin Dial 2001;14:446)

Cause: There are several clinical scenarios associated with dialysis catheter infection. *Catheter sepsis* is the most common form of catheter-related infection. It may or may not be associated with an infection at the exit site of the catheter or the subcutaneous tunnel. *Exit site infections* are characterized by erythema, tenderness, and purulent drainage in the tissue surrounding the catheter exit site. The tunnel and cuff are not involved, and there are no systemic signs of infection and no bacteremia. A tunnel infection extends along the catheter tunnel and often includes the exit site and catheter cuff. *Tunnel infections* are often accompanied by fever, systemic signs of infection, and catheter sepsis.

Epidem: Catheter sepsis episodes occur at rates of 2.0 to 5 episodes per 1000 catheter days. Exit site infections are also quite common with rates of around 2 episodes per 1000 catheter days. Tunnel infection rates are quite low at only 0.15 to 0.21 episodes per 1000 catheter days.

3% of patients with catheters will die each year due to a catheter-related infection. This is 3 times the risk of death due to infection compared to patients with an AVF or AVG (Kidney Int 2002;62:620). 50% of catheter sepsis episodes are due to Gram-positive cocci, and *Staphylococcus aureus* is the most common single organism. Gram-negative rods account for about 25% of episodes.

Pathophys: Catheter sepsis can arise from bacteria entering the hub and then growing on the luminal surface and eventually reaching the bloodstream. Bacterial adhesion properties are important in the pathogenesis of this process. Catheter sepsis can also occur when a catheter becomes infected by hematogenous spread of bacteria from another infected site.

Exit site infections arise from contamination of the exit site by pathogenic bacteria. Irritation from a tug on the catheter, a suture to secure the catheter in place, and breakdowns in hygiene are predisposing factors for this type of infection.

Tunnel infections usually start at the exit site and extend into the deep tissues to the catheter cuff and eventually to the vein. Noncuffed catheters are more prone to this type of infection.

Si:

- Fever in a dialysis patient with a catheter will turn out to be catheter sepsis 70% of the time.
- Shaking chill during dialysis.
- Tunnel infection has tenderness over the tunnel and purulent drainage.

Cmplc:

- Osteomyelitis
- Septic arthritis

- Septic pulmonary emboli
- Spinal epidural abscess
- Endocarditis

Complications are more common with *Staphylococcus aureus*.

Episodes of infection often result in missed dialysis sessions in order to get safe access.

Lab: CBCD, blood cultures

Catheter sepsis is diagnosed by positive blood cultures. Blood cultures drawn peripherally are the gold standard, but positive blood cultures drawn from the catheter or from the dialysis circuit in a patient with systemic symptoms of infection are very specific for catheter sepsis.

Exit site cultures are not helpful for diagnosis of exit site infections. The skin is not sterile, so the diagnosis is usually made on clinical grounds.

Patients with tunnel infections should also have blood cultures obtained.

Rx: Catheter sepsis and even the suspicion of catheter sepsis are indications for iv antibiotics. Once blood cultures have been obtained, the antibiotics should be infused. The initial antibiotic choice should include coverage for *Staphylococcus aureus*. A first generation cephalosporin is a good choice, but if MRSA is prevalent in the dialysis unit, vancomycin can be chosen. Patients who are acutely ill should have broader coverage to include MRSA and Gram-negative rods. A third generation cephalosporin or an aminoglycoside can be added to vancomycin as empiric coverage. Severely ill patients should be admitted to the hospital, and immediate removal of the catheter should be considered. When sepsis is confirmed, antibiotics should be switched to the narrowest coverage possible. Vancomycin should be reserved for Gram-positive bacteria that are resistant to methicillin (or patient with difficult allergies) in order to lessen the development of vancomycin-resistant enterococcus. If the organism is a Gram-negative rod or *Enterococcus*, a search for a potential genitourinary or gastrointestinal source should be undertaken.

Often the decision to continue using the catheter is made. Several observational studies have shown that antibiotics alone result in a cure in only about 30% of cases. The failures are likely due to the biofilm of bacteria in the lumen of an infected catheter. To increase the chances of cure, the catheter can be exchanged over a guidewire. Alternatively, antibiotics can be instilled in the catheter to dwell between dialysis sessions for the next 3 weeks. Vancomycin with gentamicin and vancomycin with an extended spectrum cephalosporin have been used to increase the success rate of salvaging the catheters to approximately 75%. Infection with *Staphylococcus aureus* and the presence of an exit site infection are risk factors for failure of catheter salvage. If the patient has systemic signs of infection 48 hours after antibiotics have been initiated, the catheter should be removed.

Exit site infections are treated with local skin care. Oral or iv antibiotics that cover Gram-positive cocci are usually given for 2 weeks.

Tunnel infections require immediate catheter removal and iv antibiotics. The duration of antibiotic therapy is usually 6 weeks. A new permanent catheter can be placed at a new site when the patient is free of systemic signs of sepsis.

Prevention of catheter infections is best accomplished by good catheter care.

KDOQI guidelines outline an exit site care protocol that consists of cleansing the site and the catheter with an antimicrobial solution and then dressing the site with a sterile gauze or transparent dressing material. All of this is done with aseptic technique (Am J Kidney Dis 2006;48[suppl 1]:S248).

Dialysis Catheter Thrombosis

(Semin Dial 2001;14:441)

Cause: Catheter malfunction is defined as catheter flows less than 300 ml/min during dialysis. Early catheter malfunction is usually due to malposition of the catheter tip or local swelling over the subcutaneous tunnel. Malfunction that develops 2 weeks or later after insertion is usually due to catheter thrombosis. The thrombi can be located in the catheter lumen or at the catheter tip. A fibrin sheath can also form along the outside of the catheter and interfere with blood flow. Central venous thrombosis can also cause catheter malfunction.

Epidem: Catheter failure due to poor flow is the most common cause of catheter removal. Catheter patency rates have been measured at about 80 days. The high frequency of this complication contributes to the fact that patients dialyzed with a catheter have a lower dose of dialysis compared to patients dialyzed with a fistula or graft.

Pathophys: Clots within the lumen or at the tip are likely a consequence of inadequate anticoagulation solution in the catheter between dialysis sessions. The catheter design has several outflow holes, and some of the heparin solution placed in the catheter will leak into the bloodstream after instillation. Fibrin sheath formation usually starts where the catheter enters the vein. The presence of foreign body in the vein is thrombogenic. Once the process has begun, the sheath extends along the catheter where it eventually covers the holes for inflow and outflow. Often this sheath will allow the catheter to function well for venous return of blood but not well for arterial inflow. The sheath can act as a flap that closes with the negative pressure from aspiration.

Sx: Usually none, but acute central vein thrombosis can be associated with inflammation of the vein involved and swelling of the arm or face on the same side as the catheter.

Si: Low blood flows at dialysis; increased pressure alarms at dialysis

Cmplc: Catheters with thrombosis have a higher rate of infection.

Rx: Catheter malfunction is usually treated with intraluminal instillation of thrombolytic agents. TPA is available in a 2 mg dose. Sterile water is added to make a volume equal to the catheter lumen and then instilled. The minimum dwell time is one-half hour, and it can be left to dwell until the next dialysis treatment. After the dwell, the solution is withdrawn from the catheter, and dialysis is resumed. Failures of this therapy are not uncommon, and those patients are referred for a new catheter. At the time of new catheter placement, dye should be placed into the old catheter to look for a fibrin sheath. If one is present, it should be broken up by placing a balloon over a wire into the sheath and disrupting it. Once this has been done, the new catheter can be placed over a guidewire. Central vein thrombosis is treated with catheter removal and 1 month of systemic anticoagulation.

Prevention of thrombotic complications is mainly accomplished by adequate use of anticoagulants placed in the catheter between sessions. At the end of dialysis, each port is flushed with 10 ml of sterile saline, and then a volume of heparin solution 0.1 ml larger than the lumen of the catheter is instilled to dwell until the next treatment. Systemic anticoagulation with warfarin has not proven successful for maintaining patency.

Central Venous Stenosis

Clinical Practice Guidelines for Vascular Access (Am J Kidney Dis 2006;48[suppl 1]:S248)

Cause: Central venous stenosis is a complication of catheter placement into the internal jugular and subclavian veins. Placement of pacemaker wires and peripherally inserted central catheters can also predispose a patient to develop this complication. It can even develop de novo after placement of an arteriovenous access in the ipsilateral arm.

Epidem: The subclavian veins are the most likely ones to sustain this complication. Approximately 40% of patients who have ever had a catheter placed in the subclavian vein will develop subclavian vein stenosis. The right internal jugular vein is associated with the lowest rates of venous stenosis at around 10% (Nephrol Dial Transplant 1991;6:722).

Pathophys: The foreign body in the vein causes vein wall thickening.

Si: Usually asymptomatic until an arteriovenous access is placed in the ipsilateral arm. With the increased blood flow, the obstruction can lead to arm edema and the development of dilated venous collaterals on the upper arm and chest.

Cmplc: Access thrombosis

Xray: Venography is indicated when there is massive arm edema. In addition, it is part of the workup after arteriovenous access thrombosis. Ultrasound imaging can detect the stenosis in patients who do not have arteriovenous access established.

Rx: The stenosis should be treated initially with angioplasty. Unfortunately, the likelihood of recurrence is high. If recurrences are frequent or occur in less than 3 months, a stent can be placed. Stented lesions can restenose, and in those cases you must consider ligation of the access in order to alleviate the patient's symptoms. This will require the creation of a new access.

Prevention is always preferred, and it is imperative to avoid subclavian placement of catheters in patients with CKD stage 3 or higher. The right internal jugular is the optimal site to place central venous access in this group of patients. If subclavian stenosis is detected by ultrasound prior to access creation, it is optimal to place the vascular access in the contralateral arm.

END STAGE RENAL DISEASE

9.7 Peritoneal Dialysis

Epidem: Peritoneal dialysis as a modality choice is on the decline in the United States. In 1992, 13.5% of patients who started dialysis began with peritoneal dialysis, and 14.7% of all patients receiving dialysis were on peritoneal dialysis. In 2003, only 6.9% of patients started dialysis with peritoneal dialysis, and 8.3% of all dialysis patients were using peritoneal dialysis. The number of patients on peritoneal dialysis was highest in 1995 at 30,529; by 2003 the number had fallen to 25,892. This was at a time when the total number of dialysis patients increased from 200,000 to over 300,000 (USRDS Annual Data Report, 2006).

Some of the decline is due to the fact that many more patients switch from peritoneal dialysis to hemodialysis rather than vice versa. Among the reasons for switching are inadequate dialysis, infectious complications, and patient burnout. The decline in new starts on peritoneal dialysis is hard to explain. Physician attitude surveys indicate physicians feel this modality is underutilized (Am J Kidney Dis 2001;37:22). There is no clear advantage in patient survival to either modality (Kidney Int 2006;70:S3). Patient preference may play the largest role. It is possible to reverse the decline in peritoneal dialysis as a modality choice by creating an extensive and comprehensive support unit for physicians, nurses, and patients (Adv Perit Dial 2001;17:122).

9.8 Peritoneal Dialysis Principles and Prescription

Pathophys: Peritoneal dialysis, like hemodialysis, relies on the same concepts of diffusion and ultrafiltration. The dialysate solution in this case is placed in the peritoneal cavity, and the membrane is the series of cell layers and interstitial spaces starting with the capillary endothelium and ending at the peritoneal epithelium. Over time the dialysate solution and the blood plasma approach equilibrium. The concentration gradient, dwell time, permeability of the membrane, and size of the membrane determine amount of waste products removed. The peritoneal membrane is permeable to both small- and medium-size waste products. There is also an obligate loss of protein (mainly albumin) during peritoneal dialysis. The protein loss can lead to the elimination of protein-bound waste products but also contributes to hypoalbuminemia. Ultrafiltration by peritoneal dialysis is accomplished using an osmotic pressure gradient across the peritoneum rather than a hydrostatic one. The membrane is semipermeable to glucose, so the dialysate, which contains a high concentration of glucose, will draw an ultrafiltrate into the peritoneal solution. Time is a critical factor here, because as the dwell time increases, the osmotic pressure decrease due to the influx of the ultrafiltrate and slow absorption of glucose.

The ultrafiltrate contains both water and dissolved solutes, so it also contributes to elimination of waste products. In fact, because the total volume of dialysate is much smaller than used for hemodialysis, the waste products eliminated in the ultrafiltrate can contribute significantly to the total amount of clearance.

Rx:

Peritoneal dialysis prescription
See Table 9.6.

Table 9.6   Components of a Peritoneal Dialysis Prescription

Schedule—CAPD/CCPD
Number of exchanges
Volume of exchanges
Dialysate osmotic characteristics
Dialysate electrolyte characteristics
Dwell time

- Schedule, number of exchanges, and volume of exchanges
Peritoneal dialysis is a daily procedure, but there are 2 major variations in the schedule. The simplest form is continuous ambulatory peritoneal dialysis (CAPD). The CAPD patient always has peritoneal dialysate present in the abdomen, and this fluid is exchanged several times during the day. Usually 4 exchanges are prescribed: the first daily exchange is done upon waking, another at bedtime, and the other 2 are spread out during the day. Continuous cycling peritoneal dialysis (CCPD) is performed with the assist of a cycler, which automates the exchange process. On this schedule, the bulk of dialysis is performed at night when the patient attaches the peritoneal dialysis catheter to the bags of dialysate on the cycler. The cycler uses a series of clamps to alternately fill and drain the abdomen several times each night while the patient sleeps in bed. In the morning, a final fill volume of dialysate is placed in the patient's abdomen that the patient will carry all day until he/she prepares to reattach to the cycler at night. As many as 5 cycles can be programmed for the night.

    In CAPD, the volume of all the exchanges is usually the same size. A volume of 2000 ml is well tolerated by most adult patients. Patients who are large may require 3000 ml per exchange in order to get adequate dialysis. The volumes in CCPD are often variable. The nighttime cycle volume can be individualized to provide optimal clearances. The patient's daytime volume can be very low, which maximizes comfort while ambulatory; however, if the patient requires increased clearances, larger volumes can be carried during the day, and it also is possible to schedule extra exchanges during the day.
- Dialysate osmotic characteristics
The choices for dialysate are the same for patients on CAPD or CCPD. The most common variable is the concentration of glucose (the osmotic agent) in the dialysate. The standard preparations are 1.5%, 2.5%, and 4.25%. The choice of

solution is based on the amount of ultrafiltration required to keep the patient euvolemic. There is a nonglucose osmotic agent available commercially. Icodextrin is a polymer that is not transported across the peritoneal membrane. Since the concentration is diminished only by dilution (rather than dilution and absorption for glucose), this agent is very effective for ultrafiltration in patients who do poorly with the glucose solutions (BMC Nephrol 2001;2:2).

- Dialysate electrolyte characteristics

  The electrolytes in the peritoneal dialysate are mostly standardized. The sodium concentration is 132 mEq/L. There is no potassium in the peritoneal dialysis solutions. Hypokalemia occurs in about 10% of peritoneal dialysis patients, and they are either instructed to eat a high potassium diet or given potassium supplements. There is a choice of low calcium (2.5 mEq/L) or high calcium (3.5 mEq/L) dialysate, but most patients are on low calcium dialysate to avoid calcific complications common to dialysis patients. The buffering anion is lactate because of solubility issues with solutions containing bicarbonate and calcium. This results in a bicarbonate diffusion into the dialysate and lactate diffusion into the patient. For each mmol of lactate that is absorbed, the liver will generate 1 mmol of bicarbonate. This means that patients will not develop significant acid-base disturbances due to the dialysis process.

- Dwell time

  The dwell time is an important determinant of the amount of ultrafiltration. Glucose-containing solutions have high rates of ultrafiltration the first 2 hours and then gradually fall. After 4 hours it is not uncommon for the patient to start absorbing some of the dialysate. Rapid exchanges every 1 to 2 hours can be prescribed for acute fluid overload. Icodextrin continues to maintain ultrafiltration for up to 14 hours. For patients with difficulty maintaining fluid balance with glucose-based solutions, icodextrin can be used for the long daytime dwells of patients on CCPD and the long nighttime dwells for patients on CAPD.

9.9 Peritoneal Dialysis Adequacy

Clinical Practice Guidelines for Peritoneal Dialysis Adequacy, Update 2006 (Am J Kidney Dis 2006;48[suppl 1]:S91)

Pathophys: Adequate peritoneal dialysis is defined as the dose required to optimize the patient's morbidity and mortality. The Canada-United States (CANUSA) study demonstrated that increased levels of urea clearance were associated with improvements in patient survival (J Am Soc Nephrol 1996;7:198). One important aspect of this study is that the urea clearance was measured by combining the clearance from the peritoneal dialysis process with the patients' residual kidney function (RKF). Improvements in outcome were noted up to a weekly Kt/V of 2.0. Further investigation of this data revealed that patients with the highest RKF had the best outcomes and that this confounded the data to some degree as these patients also tended to have higher weekly Kt/V values (J Am Soc Nephrol 2001;12:2158). More recent studies have shown that weekly Kt/V of 1.7 will provide optimal benefit for patients. This leads to the current KDOQI recommendation to obtain a minimum weekly Kt/V (combined peritoneal dialysis Kt/V and RKF) of 1.7 and to try to preserve the residual kidney function.

Lab: Compared to hemodialysis, it is remarkably easy to measure the dose of peritoneal dialysis using urea kinetic modeling. The urea clearance (K_{urea}) can be calculated by collecting 24 hours of the dialysate and a BUN value just as creatinine clearance can be measured with a 24-hour urine collection and a serum creatinine level.

$$K_{\text{urea peritoneal}}(\text{L/d}) = \frac{\text{Urea nitrogen (peritoneal)} \times \text{L of dialysate}}{\text{BUN} \times 1 \text{ day}}$$

To calculate the weekly Kt/V, we simply plug in 7 days for the t, and V is the volume of distribution of urea:

- V_{urea} (L) = $0.6 \times$ wt (kg) for males
- V_{urea} (L) = $0.55 \times$ wt (kg) for females

$$\text{Weekly Kt/V}_{\text{peritoneal}} = \frac{K_{\text{urea peritoneal}}(\text{L/day}) \times 7 \text{ days}}{V_{\text{urea}}(\text{L})}$$

Residual kidney function is also an important component of waste removal for patients on peritoneal dialysis. Residual kidney function is measured on all patients who produce more than 100 ml of urine in a day. To estimate the GFR in these patients with low kidney function, the GFR is calculated as the average of the creatinine clearance and urea clearance based on a 24-hour urine collection.

$$GFR(\text{L/d}) = \frac{\left(\dfrac{\text{Urine cre} \times \text{V of Urine (L/d)}}{\text{Serum Cre}}\right) + \left(\dfrac{\text{Urine urea nitrogen} \times \text{V of Urine (L/d)}}{\text{BUN}}\right)}{2}$$

To calculate the weekly clearance provided by the residual kidney function:

$$\text{Weekly Kt/V}_{\text{RKF}} = \frac{\text{GFR (L/d)} \times 7 \text{ days}}{V_{\text{urea}}(\text{L})}$$

The total weekly urea clearance is:

$$\text{Weekly Kt/V} = \text{Weekly Kt/V}_{\text{peritoneal}} + \text{Weekly Kt/V}_{\text{RKF}}$$

END STAGE RENAL DISEASE

Cmplc: Inadequate dialysis can lead to the following complications:

- Uremic manifestations
  - Decreased appetite
  - Nausea
  - Pericarditis
  - Weakness
  - Lethargy
- Fluid overload
- Increased risk of death

Rx: Peritoneal dialysis adequacy should be measured during the first 4 to 8 weeks of therapy and 4 times annually. When the dose is below the target of 1.7 or if the patient appears to have uremic manifestations, the dialysis dose should be increased. Generally, an increase in the volume of peritoneal dialysate used in a 24-hour period is prescribed. The optimal manner in which to increase the dialysis dose should be based on the patient's peritoneal membrane transport characteristics (see Peritoneal Equilibration Test). For a slow transporter, the volume of each dwell should be increased, whereas for a fast transporter, the total number of dwells each day should be increased. There are limits to what can be accomplished with peritoneal dialysis, including discomfort caused by large volume dwells or time constraints of performing multiple exchanges daily. Some patients may simply reach the limit of what they can do with this technique, and if they do not achieve adequate dialysis, they should consider a switch to hemodialysis.

Peritoneal Equilibration Test

Clinical Practice Guidelines for Peritoneal Dialysis Adequacy, Update 2006 (Am J Kidney Dis 2006;48[suppl 1]:S91)

Pathophys: The elimination of waste products with peritoneal dialysis relies on the transportation of solute across the peritoneal epithelium. This makes the peritoneal surface analogous to the hemodialysis filter. In order to appropriately prescribe and adjust the peritoneal dialysis prescription, it is important to understand the transport characteristics of this epithelial surface. The peritoneal equilibration test (PET) measures the transport of glucose and creatinine across the peritoneal epithelium. The test results are obtained at the end of a 4-hour dwell with 2000 ml of a 2.5% glucose solution. The final concentration of glucose and creatinine in the dialysate are measured along with a serum creatinine level.

- D0 glucose = initial concentration of dialysate glucose (2500 mg/dL for a 2.5% solution)
- D glucose = final dialysate glucose concentration
- D creatinine = final dialysate creatinine concentration
- P creatinine = plasma creatinine level (usually serum level is substituted)
- The final drain volume is also measured.

D/D0 glucose represents the fraction of glucose absorption

D/P creatinine represents the solute transport of creatinine

Large studies have established mean values for D/D0 glucose at 0.38 and D/P creatinine at 0.65 (Blood Purif 1989;7:95). The majority of patients are average transporters, 15% are in the high category, and another 15% are low transporters (see Table 9.7).

Drain volumes tend to be higher with low transporters and lower with high transporters, but the drain volume is not used to define the transport status of peritoneal epithelium.

Table 9.7   Interpretation of PET Results

	D/D0 Glucose	D/P Creatinine
Average transporter	0.26–0.49	0.5–0.8
Low transporter	> 0.49	< 0.5
High transporter	< 0.26	> 0.8

END STAGE RENAL DISEASE

Cmplc: During peritonitis episodes, the inflammation of the peritoneal epithelium causes a significant increase in solute transplant. A PET should not be done until about 1 month has elapsed since a peritonitis episode. The development of intra-abdominal adhesions can reduce the solute transport rate due to a smaller surface area available for dialysis.

Lab: It is advised to perform a baseline PET approximately 4 weeks after initiation of peritoneal dialysis therapy. Follow-up PETs are indicated to investigate causes of underdialysis or poor ultrafiltration.

Rx: Low transporters should have regimens with longer dwell times. High transporters should have regimens with short dwell times. Since most regimens include at least 1 long dwell (nighttime for CAPD or daytime for CCPD), the use of icodextrin for the long dwell can improve clearance and ultrafiltration for high transporters.

9.10 Peritoneal Dialysis Complications

Peritoneal Dialysis Peritonitis

Peritoneal Dialysis-related Infections Recommendations: 2005 Update (Perit Dial Int 2005;25:107)

Cause: There are several potential routes of entry into the abdominal cavity for pathogenic bacteria. The most common route is via the lumen of the peritoneal catheter. Any break in sterile technique can introduce bacteria into the catheter lumen, which are then flushed into the peritoneal cavity. In addition, a biofilm on the inside of the catheter is an important cause of recurrent peritonitis. Bacteria can also enter the peritoneal cavity around the outside of the catheter as it traverses from the skin to the peritoneum. In these cases, an exit site infection or tunnel infection is also present. Bacteria can migrate from the intestinal tract either transmurally or from a perforation. Severe constipation and colitis are associated with peritonitis from bowel organisms. Hematogenous spread is a rare cause of peritonitis.

Epidem: Peritonitis episodes occur at a rate of about 0.5 episodes annually per patient at risk. Exit site infections are concurrent in approximately 20% of them. Whether the method of peritoneal dialysis, either CAPD or CCPD, is associated with a lower risk is debatable. The only data comparing peritonitis rates with different methods are from retrospective observational studies. An evaluation of United States Medicare patients from 1994 to 1997 revealed a rate of 0.53 episodes annually per patient on CCPD compared to 0.50 episodes annually per patient on CAPD (Am J Kidney Dis 2005;45:372).

The microbiology of most peritonitis episodes indicates they are due to entrance of the bacteria into the peritoneal cavity from the skin (see Table 9.8).

Pathophys: It is obvious that the peritoneal dialysis catheter circumvents host defenses by breaking the physical barrier of the peritoneal epithelium and also provides a direct route for bacteria to enter the abdomen through its lumen. The peritoneal dialysate also is a contributing factor. Characteristics of the peritoneal dialysate that impair macrophage function are the high glucose concentration and acidic pH. The glucose content also provides an excellent growth medium.

END STAGE RENAL DISEASE

Table 9.8   Microbiology of Peritoneal Dialysis Peritonitis

Gram-positive organisms	67%
Gram-negative organisms	28%
Polymicrobial	15%
Fungal	2.5%
Culture negative	20%

(Am J Kidney Dis 2000;36:1009)

During an episode of peritonitis, the inflamed peritoneal membrane will have altered transport characteristics. Solute transport increases and ultrafiltration decreases, and there is an increased loss of albumin into the dialysate.

Si: Cloudy dialysis fluid and abdominal pain are presumed to be due to peritonitis.

Sx: Abdominal tenderness with or without rebound tenderness, fever, hypotension

Cmplc: Peritonitis is the leading cause for patients to switch to hemodialysis. 15% of cases result in catheter removal. Peritonitis is associated with an overall increase in mortality for patients on peritoneal dialysis. It is estimated that a rise in peritonitis rate by 0.5% annually will be associated with a 10% increase in all cause mortality. Mortality is not just due to death as a complication of the peritonitis but also from the malnutrition and potential inadequate dialysis that accompany many episodes of peritonitis (J Am Soc Nephrol 1996;7:2176).

Lab:

- Peritoneal fluid studies
  - Cell count and diff
  - Gram stain
  - Culture
    WBC > $100/mm^3$ with more than 50% polys is enough evidence to initiate treatment.
- Blood tests
  - CBCD
  - Blood cultures

Xray: CT scan of the abdomen and pelvis can be done if perforation is suspected.

Rx: Because of the poor outcomes and increased mortality associated with peritonitis in peritoneal dialysis patients, the International

Society for Peritoneal Dialysis has published a set of guidelines that have a strong focus on prevention as well as treatment.

Prevention:

- Perioperative antibiotics should be administered at the time of catheter insertion.
- Exit site care is critical (see Peritoneal Dialysis Catheter Exit Site and Tunnel Infection).
- Extensive patient training in sterile technique is associated with lower rates of peritonitis.
- Programs should perform outcomes monitoring. If a program has a rate greater than 0.67 episodes annually per patient, a performance improvement plan should be initiated to obtain a goal less than 0.5 episodes annually.

Therapy: Initial antibiotic coverage is empiric to cover both Gram-positive and Gram-negative organisms. In the rare case that the Gram stain is helpful, the coverage can be narrowed according to the Gram stain results. Gram-positive coverage is provided by vancomycin or first generation cephalosporins. The decision to choose vancomycin over a cephalosporin should be based on the program's rate of methicillin-resistant Gram-positive organisms. Gram-negatives are covered by a third generation cephalosporin or an aminoglycoside. The preferred route of delivery is via the intraperitoneal route. Dosing can be either continuous or daily for cephalosporins and aminoglycosides or intermittent for vancomycin. If once daily or intermittent dosing is used, the dwell time should be 6 hours for the exchange that contains antibiotics (see Table 9.9).

In over 80% of cases, the cultures will be positive within 72 hours. Further antibiotic therapy should be based on the organism.

- Coagulase negative staphylococci: Antibiotic choice should be based on sensitivities. This organism is often methicillin resistant, so vancomycin therapy is required. The infection can

Table 9.9 Common Antibiotic Regimens for Peritoneal Dialysis Peritonitis

Antibiotic	Intermittent dosing (1 exchange)	Continuous dosing
Vancomycin	15–30 mg/kg every 5–7 days redose when serum level < 15 mcg/ml	LD 1000 mg/L MD 25 mg/L
Gentamicin	0.6 mg/kg daily	LD 8 mg/L MD 4 mg/L
Cefazolin	15 mg/kg daily	LD 500 mg/L MD 125 mg/L
Ceftazidime	1000–1500 mg daily	LD 500 mg/L MD 125 mg/L

LD = loading dose in 2000 ml exchange; MD = maintenance dose (in every exchange)

usually be resolved with a 2-week course of antibiotics. Recurrent infection with this organism can indicate a pathogenic biofilm in the catheter. Catheter removal is advised under those circumstances.

- Streptococci and enterococci: Ampicillin is the drug of choice for these infections. Continuous therapy with 125 mg added to each L of dialysate is the recommended dose. Severe infections should be treated for 3 weeks. Vancomycin is used if sensitivities indicate ampicillin resistance.

- *Staphylococcus aureus*: *Staphylococcus aureus* infection should be treated for 3 weeks with the appropriate antibiotic based on sensitivities. A tunnel infection should be searched for very diligently as the combination of a tunnel infection and peritonitis will require catheter removal for definitive treatment.

- *Pseudomonas aeruginosa*: *Pseudomonas aeruginosa* infection is also often associated with a tunnel infection, and likewise, catheter removal will be required if that is the case. To treat an isolated *Pseudomonas aeruginosa* infection requires the use of 2 antibiotics; an oral quinolone combined with an antipseudomonal cephalosporin or aminoglycoside are good options. 3 weeks of therapy are advised.

- Single Gram-negative organism: These are treated with a single antibiotic based on sensitivity. Outcomes are generally worse than infections with single Gram-positive organisms with respect to death and catheter loss. 3 weeks of therapy are advised.

- Polymicrobial: Culture of multiple enteric organisms suggests an intestinal perforation as the cause, and a surgical evaluation is warranted. Triple antibiotic regimens to cover Gram-negative, Gram-positive, and anaerobic organisms are advised. For example, metronidazole, ampicillin, and a third generation cephalosporin or aminoglycoside. Culture of multiple Gram-positive organisms suggests infection introduced through the lumen, and usually a single antibiotic regimen can be employed.

- Fungal: Fungal infections require catheter removal. Appropriate antibiotic coverage should continue for 10 days after catheter removal.

- Culture negative: Culture negative peritonitis occurs in less than 20% of peritonitis episodes. If after 3 days the cultures are negative, another sample of peritoneal fluid should be sent for cell count and culture. If the cell counts are declining and the cultures remain negative, the peritonitis is resolving. Therapy with antibiotics should continue for 2 weeks. If the peritonitis is not resolving, special cultures for fungi, mycobacteria, and other pathogens should be undertaken. Infections not resolved in 5 days should be treated like a refractory peritonitis with catheter removal.

- Refractory peritonitis: Peritonitis usually responds quickly to antibiotic therapy. For patients who have not made a significant improvement within 72 hours, repeat cell counts and cultures should be obtained. If after 5 days on the appropriate antibiotic regimen there is no resolution, the catheter should be removed.

Peritoneal Dialysis Catheter Exit Site and Tunnel Infection

Peritoneal Dialysis-related Infections Recommendations: 2005 Update (Perit Dial Int 2005;25:107)

Cause: Exit site infections can result from any trauma to the area of catheter insertion, such as a tug on the catheter. They also occur in patients who develop an intense inflammatory foreign body reaction to the catheter. Tunnel infections are often preceded by exit site infections with *Staphylococcus aureus* or *Pseudomonas aeruginosa*.

Epidem: Patients with nasal carriage of *Staphylococcus aureus* often have colonization of the exit site.

Sx: Many tunnel and exit site infections are asymptomatic. Pain at the exit site or pain at the exit site and along the tunnel can be present.

Si: The hallmark of an exit site infection is purulent drainage; however, it can be difficult to distinguish reactive inflammation from an early exit site infection. Other signs of an exit site infection include edema, erythema, and crusting. Follow-up exam after intensified local cleansing and re-education about strategies to secure the catheter to prevent tugs are often appropriate. A tunnel infection presents with tenderness and redness along the tunnel and purulent drainage from the tunnel.

Lab: Gram stain and culture of purulent drainage

Xray: Ultrasonography of the tunnel can be used to diagnose a suspected tunnel infection.

Rx: In cases where no cultures are performed or before culture results are available, empiric coverage for *Staphylococcus aureus* is indicated. A first generation cephalosporin given via the oral route is a good choice. Intraperitoneal administration is an alternative. Therapy should continue for at least 2 weeks or longer if the infection has not resolved. If culture results indicate

Pseudomonas aeruginosa, an oral quinolone is appropriate. If the infection does not resolve, intraperitoneal administration of an antipseudomonal cephalosporin can be added. When there is a tunnel infection associated with peritonitis, catheter removal is required.

Prevention of exit site infections is accomplished with meticulous exit site care. Each institution should develop a strategy for daily cleansing and dressing. There are a variety of choices including soap and water, saline washes, antibacterial soaps, and antibacterial creams.

Peritoneal Membrane Failure

Cause: Peritoneal membrane failure can present with ultrafiltration failure or inadequate solute removal, resulting in inadequate dialysis. Acute causes of peritoneal membrane failure include peritonitis, outflow problems such as catheter migration, and dialysate leaks. A gradual decline in ultrafiltration is a consequence of long-term peritoneal dialysis (Kidney Int 2004;66:2437). It eventually results in discontinuation of the method in 50% of patients on peritoneal dialysis for over 6 years (Kidney Int 1998;54:2207). Inadequate solute removal is seen in sclerosing peritonitis. Other conditions that present with inadequate solute removal with normal peritoneal membrane function include patient noncompliance and loss of residual kidney function.

Pathophys: The insidious onset of ultrafiltration failure is due to enhanced solute permeability. The enhanced absorption of glucose causes a decline in the osmotic gradient responsible for ultrafiltration. Histological examination of the peritoneal membrane shows increases in vascularity. It is postulated that the chronic exposure to hyperglycemic solution leads to local accumulation of advanced glycosylation end products. These can cause a variety of effects including vasodilation, increased permeability, and angiogenesis (Perit Dial Int 2003;23[suppl 2]:S14).

END STAGE RENAL DISEASE

Sclerosing peritonitis is characterized by thick sclerotic tissue involving the peritoneal wall with or without adhesions. Chemical irritants introduced into the peritoneum, severe peritonitis, and incompletely treated peritonitis are all predisposing factors.

Sx: Inadequate solute removal may present with uremic symptomatology.

Si: Edema and poorly controlled hypertension are findings consistent with ultrafiltration failure.

Lab: When membrane failure is suspected, a PET and determination of peritoneal dialysis adequacy are indicated (see section 9.9). Cell count and culture can be ordered to rule out peritonitis.

Xray: An abdominal flat plate and a CT scan of the abdomen and pelvis may be helpful for diagnosing acute causes of membrane failure. Sclerosing peritonitis findings on CT scan include calcification and thickening of the peritoneum and loculated fluid collections.

Rx: A normal PET (or one unchanged from the patient's baseline) suggests either noncompliance with the prescribed regimen or loss of residual kidney function. Measurement of peritoneal dialysis adequacy can usually sort those out. An increase in peritoneal dialysis regimen or change in modality is often required when the residual kidney function declines. The long-term peritoneal dialysis patient with ultrafiltration failure and a PET demonstrating increased solute transport can continue peritoneal dialysis with the use of a cycler set to dwell times of less than 2 hours and icodextrin for the long dwell period (Perit Dial Int 2006;26:336). When the PET demonstrates decreased solute transport, it is often inevitable to require a switch to hemodialysis. In some cases, the patient can resume peritoneal dialysis after a 2-month period to allow the peritoneum to heal.

Acute Outflow Problems

Cause: An abrupt decrease in peritoneal fluid volume is usually the sign of a technical problem with the catheter. Catheter migration, where the catheter moves out of the pelvis and into the mid or upper peritoneal cavity, is a common cause. A fibrin plug within the catheter lumen or wrapping of the tip in omental fat can also be responsible. Internal dialysate leaks and ultrafiltration failure can rarely present with acute change in outflow but usually are more chronic in nature.

Epidem: Constipation may predispose to omental wrapping and catheter migration. Observation of fibrin in the effluent means the patient is at risk for developing a fibrin clot in the catheter.

Sx: After the catheter migrates, the patient may no longer note a tugging sensation in the lower abdomen at the end of a drain. The patient may note the sensation is now higher in the abdomen.

Lab: If there is not a technical reason for the outflow failure, a PET can diagnose ultrafiltration failure.

Xray: A flat plate of the abdomen is indicated to locate the catheter tip. If no cause is found, a CT scan of the abdomen and pelvis can be used to look for an internal leak.

Rx: There are several approaches to get a catheter to move back into the pelvis. Stimulation of peristalsis is often successful. Ingestion of 1 gallon of polyethylene glycol electrolyte solution is an effective choice. If this fails, laparoscopic manipulation or fluoroscopic repositioning with a guidewire can be performed (Perit Dial Int 2006;26:374). Catheter migration can be prevented by placing a stitch connecting the end of the catheter to the pelvic peritoneum (Perit Dial Int 2007;27:554). A fibrin plug may be able to be dislodged with a forceful flush of 10 ml of sterile saline. Other noninvasive treatments include the addition of heparin at 500 units/L to the dialysate. TPA at a dose of 2 mg in 30 to 40 ml of saline can be instilled in the catheter for 2 hours (Adv Perit

Dial 2001;17:249). To prevent fibrin plugs, heparin (500 unit/L) should be added to the dialysate when fibrin strands are noted.

Hernias in Peritoneal Dialysis Patients

(Adv Perit Dial 2003;19:130)

Cause: The addition of peritoneal dialysate to the abdomen increases intra-abdominal pressure and predisposes peritoneal dialysis patients to hernias. Hernia locations include pericatheter, inguinal, umbilical, and previous surgical incisions.

Pathophys: Factors that contribute to increased intra-abdominal pressures include the quantity of dialysate and an upright position.

Epidem: Observational studies show that approximately 25% of peritoneal dialysis patients develop hernias. Polycystic kidney disease is a risk factor (Perit Dial Int 2003;23:249).

Sx: Pain

Si: Hernias are usually palpable on physical exam.

Xray: In obese patients, small hernias in the anterior abdominal wall may not be easily palpated. An abdominal CT scan may be necessary for diagnosis.

Rx: Hernias generally respond well to surgical correction. It is optimal to stop peritoneal dialysis for 4 weeks after the surgery. For patients prone to recurrent hernias, a peritoneal dialysis regimen of nighttime cycling in the supine position with as small a daytime dwell as possible is a recommended strategy.

Peritoneal Dialysate Leak

(Semin Dial 2001;14:50)

Cause: Peritoneal dialysate leaks can be either internal or external. Internal leaks can communicate with the retroperitoneal space, the thorax, or a hernia sac. Patients who have undergone nephrectomy have a compromised peritoneal barrier and may develop a retroperitoneal leak. Pleural leaks into the thorax are due to congenital defects in the diaphragm but also can be seen after cardiovascular surgery. External leaks occur at the catheter insertion site and are due to initiation of peritoneal dialysis prior to complete healing of the surgical incision. If the outer surgical incision is fully healed but the site of entry into the peritoneum is not secure, a leak will develop along the catheter tract and present with lower abdominal and scrotal or labial edema.

Epidem: Risk factors for the development of external or internal pericatheter dialysate leaks include older age and higher BMI (Perit Dial Int 2003;23:249).

Sx: Often asymptomatic, on occasion the swelling can cause discomfort. A pleural leak can cause dyspnea.

Si: External leaks are diagnosed by observing wetness or drainage around the exit site—generally not purulent. Dullness to percussion and decreased breath sounds signify a pleural effusion if there is a leak in the thorax. Anterior abdominal wall edema and scrotal or labial edema are signs of an internal pericatheter leak. Any internal leak may be responsible for decreased ultrafiltration or outflow failure. In fact, those features may be the only clues that there is a retroperitoneal leak.

Lab: One diagnostic feature of leaks is the high glucose content of any leaking fluid. A urinalysis test strip will read 2+ or higher. Pleural fluid glucose values of 300 mg/dL or higher are indicative of pleural leak.

Xray: CXR should be performed when there are physical exam signs of a pleural leak. A CT scan of the abdomen and pelvis can locate fluid in the retroperitoneum and any hernia sacs.

Rx: When a leak is suspected, an initial trial off peritoneal dialysis is suggested. Usually this period lasts 2 to 4 weeks. This often will lead to resolution of any symptoms and signs and the patient can resume peritoneal dialysis. If there is an external leak, a 2-week course of empiric antibiotics is advised, as there is a risk of developing a tunnel infection or peritonitis. The antibiotics should cover *Staphylococcus aureus*. Most external leaks and leaks around the catheter tract will resolve with rest. Hernias should be repaired to eliminate leaks into hernia sacs. Pleural leaks due to cardiovascular surgery also eventually seal. Congenital defects in the diaphragm usually do not resolve and require a permanent change to hemodialysis. Retroperitoneal leaks have a variable prognosis, and if they recur after a trial period off peritoneal dialysis, the patient should make a permanent switch to hemodialysis.

9.11 Nutritional Issues in the End Stage Renal Disease Patient

(Am J Kidney Dis 2005;46:371)

Cause: Maintenance of optimal nutrition is a challenge for dialysis patients. They need to achieve appropriate intake of calories and protein while limiting intake of sodium, potassium, phosphorous, and fluid. The recommended daily calorie intake is 35 kcal/kg for dialysis patients under 60 years of age and 30 to 35 kcal/kg for patients over 60 years old. The recommended daily protein intake is 1.2 g/kg.

A number of factors are responsible for inadequate nutritional intake.

- Uremia
- Inadequate dialysis
- Gastroparesis
- Inflammation
- Depression
- Poverty

Nutritional requirements in dialysis patients are elevated due to loss of nutrients into the dialysate. Water-soluble vitamins and amino acids are able to pass through the hemodialysis

Table 9.10   Dietary Restrictions for Dialysis Patients

Nutrient	Daily Restriction
Sodium	2000–4000 mg
Potassium	2000 mg
Phosphorous	1000 mg
Fluid	1 L + daily urine volume

filter. Peritoneal dialysis patients lose several grams of albumin each day into the peritoneal effluent. Another nutritional stress common in dialysis patients is increased catabolism. This is a consequence of metabolic acidosis and inflammatory states (see Table 9.10).

Patients with diabetes and/or lipid disorders may have even more limitations placed on intake.

Epidem: There are high rates of malnutrition in dialysis patient when serum albumin is used as a marker. As many as 70% of patients have albumin levels below 4.0 g/dL. For every 1 g/dL decline in serum albumin, there is a 10% increase in mortality. A BMI of less than 18.5 is also associated with increased mortality (Am J Kidney Dis 1998;31:997).

Lab: Serum albumin should be measured monthly for all patients in the dialysis unit.

Rx: Because of the serious consequences of malnutrition, nutritional assessment and treatment are an important part of managing dialysis patients. A registered dietitian is a vital member of the multidisciplinary team that cares for patients in the dialysis unit. The dietitian is responsible for an initial nutritional assessment that includes the current nutritional status. Components of the assessment should include the serum albumin, BMI, determination of ideal body weight, current dietary habits, recent weight change, and gastrointestinal symptoms such as nausea, vomiting, and anorexia. The nutritional assessment should also identify any medical, economic, or social barriers to inappropriate or inadequate nutrient intake. The final component of the assessment is to define the goals for therapy in terms of protein and calorie intake, weight gain or loss, and individualized daily limitations of sodium, potassium, phosphorous, and fluid.

See Tables 9.11 and 9.12 for a partial list of foods with high levels of potassium and phosphorous that should be limited or avoided.

An important part of the strategy to achieve these goals is nutritional counseling and monthly monitoring of the patient's nutritional status, performed by the dietitian. Nutritional

Table 9.11   Common High-Potassium Foods

Dairy products
Citrus fruits
Bananas
Melons
Dried fruits
Potatoes
Tomatoes and tomato-based products
Winter squash

Table 9.12   Common High-Phosphorous Foods

Dairy products
Whole grain products
Dark sodas
Nuts and seeds (including peanuts)
Chocolate
Dried beans and peas
Organ meats

counseling is indicated for all patients. For patients who do not meet food intake goals, there are several nutritional supplements designed specifically for dialysis patients. These supplements have a high protein content while limiting the amount of sodium, potassium, and phosphorous. They are available in powder, liquid, or solid form. Parenteral nutrition can be administered during a hemodialysis treatment by infusing nutrients into the blood returning from the dialyzer. This is called *intradialytic parenteral nutrition*. A course of IDPN results in an increase in serum albumin concentration, but no studies have established an improvement in clinical outcomes. Use of the therapy is expensive and controversial. A number of medications to treat malnutrition have been reported: megestrol acetate, human growth hormone, and anabolic steroids. Megestrol acetate is a steroid derived appetite stimulant. Trials were notable for a large number of side effects, and there is concern that it predisposes patients to thrombosis. Trials with human growth hormone have not resulted in any long-term improvement in outcomes. For the use of anabolic steroids, there are concerns about long-term and short-term adverse effects. These include personality changes, lower HDL levels, and hypercoagulability.

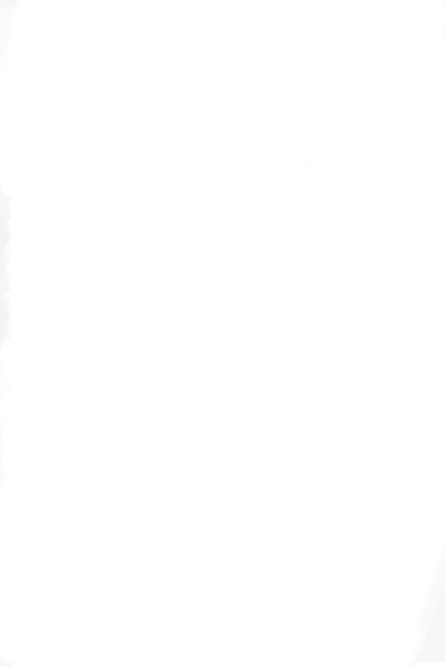

Chapter 10

Hypertension

10.1 Approach to a Patient with Hypertension

Introduction: In 2003, the Seventh Report of the Joint National Committee on Prevention, Detection, Evaluation and Treatment of High Blood Pressure (JNC 7) was published to provide an evidence-based approach to the diagnosis, treatment, and prevention of hypertension and its consequences (Hypertension 2003;42:1206).

Cause:

- Primary or essential hypertension
- Secondary hypertension (identifiable causes of hypertension)
  - Kidney disease: Renovascular hypertension; renal parenchymal disease
  - Endocrine causes: Primary hyperaldosteronism; Cushing's disease or other corticosteroid excess; pheochromocytoma; hyperthyroidism; hypothyroidism; hyperparathyroidism
  - Coarctation of the aorta
  - Sleep apnea

Epidem: Primary or essential hypertension accounts for 90% to 95% of patients with hypertension. It is estimated that 50 million people in the United States have hypertension. Worldwide, there may be 1 billion people with elevated blood pressure. The prevalence of hypertension increases strikingly with age so that more than half of people aged 60 to 69 have hypertension and, approximately 75% of the population over 70 years of age is affected.

There are also race and gender differences, with higher prevalence rates in blacks and males. A family history of hypertension is also an important risk factor. Potentially modifiable risk factors:

- Obesity
- Sedentary lifestyle
- Excessive alcohol consumption
- Smoking
- Stress
- Excessive salt intake

Pathophys: For the overwhelming majority of hypertensives who have essential hypertension, the exact pathophysiology remains unknown; however, many factors that influence the blood pressure are known. The blood pressure is a function of cardiac output and vascular resistance. The cardiac output is increased by stimuli from the sympathetic nervous system and by intravascular volume expansion. Vascular resistance is either increased or decreased by a myriad of factors that control the vascular tone in the small arterioles.

Factors that increase vascular tone:

- Angiotensin II
- Endothelin
- Calcium
- Vasopressin
- Epinephrine and norepinephrine

Factors that decrease vascular tone:

- Nitric oxide
- Prostacyclin
- Bradykinin

Physical characteristics of the small arterioles, including wall stiffness and lumen diameter, also play a role in determining vascular resistance.

Intravascular volume expansion is an important factor because it influences both the cardiac output and the vascular tone. Intravascular volume expansion increases vascular tone by expanding the vessel diameter, which in turn increases luminal pressure and wall tension (LaPlace's law). It increases cardiac output by increasing the cardiac preload.

The intravascular volume is regulated by a number of different factors:

- Sodium intake will result in intravascular volume expansion.
- Aldosterone expands the intravascular volume by decreasing sodium excretion.
- Atrial natriuretic peptide acts to decrease the intravascular volume by enhancing sodium excretion.

Many of the therapies for hypertension are directed at altering one or more aspects of this complex system.

Sx: Usually none, some patients may have headaches or nocturia.

Si: Hypertension may be the most clinically significant condition that is diagnosed solely on the basis of physical exam findings. Accurate measurement of the blood pressure is critical to making the diagnosis (see section 10.3 and Table 10.1).

Table 10.1 JNC 7 Blood Pressure Classification

	Systolic Blood Pressure		Diastolic Blood Pressure
Normal	< 120 mm Hg	and	< 80 mm Hg
Prehypertension	120–139 mm Hg	or	80–89 mm Hg
Stage 1 hypertension	140–159 mm Hg	or	90–99 mm Hg
Stage 2 hypertension	≥ 160 mm Hg	or	≥ 100 mm Hg

Cmplc: Hypertension is a risk factor for damage to a number of organ systems.

- Cardiac
  - Coronary artery disease
  - Congestive heart failure
  - Left ventricular hypertrophy
- Kidney
  - Nephrosclerosis
  - Progression of CKD due to any diagnosis
- CNS
  - Hemorrhagic stroke
  - Ischemic stroke
  - Dementia
  - Macular degeneration
- Peripheral arterial disease
- Erectile dysfunction

Lab: Several tests are usually done on all new hypertensives in order to make a cursory screen for secondary causes, to assess any potential end organ damage, and to evaluate other cardiac risk factors.

- Serum potassium to look for potential high aldosterone states that would present with hypokalemia.
- Estimated GFR and urinalysis to screen for CKD either as a cause or as end organ damage.
- Glucose and lipids are typically checked as part of completing the cardiac risk factor analysis.
- EKG can be done to screen for coronary artery disease and left ventricular hypertrophy.

Rx: The target blood pressure for most patients with hypertension is 140/90 mm Hg. In patients with diabetes or CKD, the target blood pressure is lower (see section 10.12).

In order to reach goal, patients need a combination of lifestyle modifications and medications. The lifestyle modifications include weight loss for overweight patients and reduction in daily sodium intake to approx 2.4 g (100 mmol). The adoption of the Dietary Approach to Stop Hypertension (DASH) diet, which is high in fruits, vegetables, low fat dairy products, and low in cholesterol will assist in blood pressure control. Regular aerobic exercise is indicated for patients who are capable, and ethanol intake should be no more than 1 oz (30 ml) daily.

The majority of patients will not meet goal with attempts at lifestyle modifications, so they will need to initiate medication therapy. The initial choice of medication therapy is based on the stage of hypertension and the presence of any conditions that would provide compelling indications for individual drug classes (see Table 10.2).

Patients without compelling indications and stage 1 hypertension should be started on a thiazide diuretic. Other agents that could be considered for initial therapy are ACEIs, ARBs, beta blockers, or calcium channel blockers. If a single agent fails to control blood pressure, an agent from another class should be added. Patients with stage 2 hypertension should be placed on a 2-drug regimen with a thiazide diuretic and ACEI, ARB, beta blocker, or calcium channel blocker. Follow-up visits are usually monthly while the blood pressure is not under control.

Table 10.2   Choice of Initial Antihypertensive Medication Agent Based on Compelling Indications

Compelling Indication	Initial Antihypertensive Agent
Ischemic heart disease	Beta blocker
Heart failure	ACEI or ARB
Diabetes mellitus	ACEI or ARB
CKD	ACEI or ARB
Cerebrovascular disease	ACEI and a diuretic

For patients with the compelling indication of ischemic heart disease, beta blockers are usually part of the regimen. For patients with heart failure, diabetes, or CKD, the initial therapy should include ACEI or ARB. For patients with previous cerebrovascular disease, the combination of ACEI and a diuretic has been shown to reduce the occurrence of recurrent stroke.

10.2 Hypertension in the Community

Epidem: The prevention of hypertension presents a major public health challenge. The prevalence of lifestyle risk factors, such as obesity, physical inactivity, and excess sodium intake, are all very high. Since the genesis and cultivation of these occur in the community, it is likely that the interventions must take place there. Community-based proposals to decrease these risk factors include lobbying the food industry to reduce sodium content, providing more places to engage in physical activity, and promoting healthy food choices in schools and workplaces (JAMA 2002;288:1882).

Crs:
(Hypertension 2003;42:1206)
According to the JNC 7 report, over the past 30 years the awareness of hypertension has increased from 51% of patients in the period 1976 to 1980 to 70% in 1999 to 2000. The percentage of hypertensives receiving treatment increased from 31% to 59% in the same period. Between 1960 and 1991, the median systolic blood pressure for individuals from ages 61 to 74 declined by 16 mm Hg. Improved management of hypertension is likely responsible for some of the 60% decline in mortality from cerebrovascular disease and 50% decline in mortality due to CAD seen since 1972.

Rx: The number of patients who meet goals for treatment of their hypertension is only 34% according to the JNC 7 report. Patient nonadherence and provider behavior play significant roles in the failure to achieve goals. The failure to intensify or initiate therapy during a physician visit when the blood pressure goal has not been reached is termed clinical inertia. The reasons for clinical inertia are felt to be overestimation of care given, use of "soft" indications to avoid intensification of therapy, and lack of training and practice organization based on goals (Ann Intern Med 2001;135:825). Automated reminder systems, practice report cards, and even "pay for performance" are potential solutions to overcome clinical inertia (Curr Hypertens Rep 2006;8:324). Strategies to improve patient adherence include patient education, improved patient–physician communication, increased clinic hours, and uncomplicated dosing schedules.

10.3   Blood Pressure Measurement

(Hypertension 2005;45:142)

Epidem: The physician's office is the traditional location to diagnose and monitor the treatment of hypertension. Ambulatory and home blood pressure readings can be useful for these purposes as well. It is becoming increasingly common to find automated blood pressure devices in public places. As of 1995, over 10 million measurements were made by these machines yearly. The proliferation of blood pressure measurement devices available for the consumer testifies to the popularity of self-blood pressure measurement in the home. The blood pressure levels for diagnosing hypertension and assessing blood pressure control with ambulatory and home readings are lower than the criteria used in the office setting (see Table 10.3).

Many blood pressure readings are part of the patient's vital signs (eg, in the emergency room or during a dialysis treatment). These measurements are made in clinical settings and with techniques that are often distinct from those used to diagnose hypertension.

Table 10.3 Criteria for Normal Blood Pressure and Blood Pressure Control* in Different Settings

Setting	Systolic Blood Pressure		Diastolic Blood Pressure
Office-based normal	< 130 mm Hg	and	< 80 mm Hg
Home or ambulatory normal	< 125 mm Hg	and	< 75 mm Hg
Office-based goal	< 140 mm Hg	and	< 90 mm Hg
Home or ambulatory goal	< 135 mm Hg	and	< 85 mm Hg

*nondiabetic, no CKD

Pathophys: There are several noninvasive methods used to measure the blood pressure.

The *auscultatory method* has been in use for over 100 years. It is based on the appearance and disappearance of the Korotkoff sounds. These sounds are heard over the brachial artery during gradual decompression of the vessel after it has been occluded proximally by a cuff. The appearance of the first sound corresponds to the systolic blood pressure. The disappearance of the final sound corresponds to the diastolic blood pressure.

In order to assure accurate readings, a well trained observer and a calibrated device are important. Important aspects of observer training include gradual decompression of the cuff at a rate of 2 mm Hg/sec and estimation of blood pressure to the nearest 2 mm Hg. Several kinds of devices are available. The traditional device is the mercury sphygmomanometer. This device is quite accurate but creates obvious environmental concerns. The most common device in use is the aneroid sphygmomanometer. There are many manufacturers of these devices, and it is important to choose a high quality model if you are going to use one to diagnose and treat hypertension. These devices should also be tested for accuracy on a regular basis.

The *oscillometric technique* is employed by most automated blood pressure measurement devices. It is based on oscillations of pressure that occur during gradual decompression of an artery that has been occluded by a sphygmomanometer cuff. The oscillations are maximal at mean arterial pressure but start at pressures higher than the systolic and end at pressures lower than diastolic blood pressure. During cuff deflation, the machine registers the magnitude of the oscillations and uses an algorithm to determine the systolic and diastolic blood pressures. Each device contains an algorithm that is proprietary to the device manufacturer. The accuracy of these machines corresponds well to the auscultatory method and intra-arterial blood pressure measurement.

Rx: The final component to assuring accurate office-based pressure measurement is a well-prepared patient. The correct size blood pressure cuff should be used (see Table 10.4).

The cuff should be placed on the bare arm of the patient. The sleeve should not be rolled up as it could create a tourniquet effect. The patient's arm should be supported and raised to the level of the heart so that the cuff is level with the approximate location of the right atrium. The patient should be seated with the back supported and the legs uncrossed. Five minutes of quiet time prior to blood pressure measurement is appropriate to allow the patient to relax.

Table 10.4   Recommended Blood Pressure Cuff Sizes

Arm Circumference	Size	Cuff Dimensions
22–26 cm	Small adult	12 cm × 22 cm
27–34 cm	Adult	16 cm × 30 cm
35–44 cm	Large adult	16 cm × 36 cm
45–52 cm	Adult thigh	16 cm × 42 cm

For patients who want to purchase a home blood pressure monitor, the dabl Educational Trust (www.dableducational.org) is a good resource to look for a device that has been validated for accuracy. Care must be taken with blood pressure monitoring devices that measure the blood pressure at the wrist in order to place the limb in the correct position so the cuff is at the same level as the right atrium. Finger blood pressure devices are not recommended because of limb position problems and peripheral vasoconstriction.

10.4   White Coat Hypertension

Cause:

White coat hypertension: Patients who consistently meet criteria for the diagnosis of hypertension when their blood pressure is measured at the office but have normal blood pressure in the ambulatory setting.

White coat effect: Patients who have been diagnosed with hypertension that do not meet goal with office based readings but meet targets based on ambulatory measurements (see section 10.6).

These phenomena are believed to be due to anxiety associated with visiting a physician's office.

Epidem: Among patients who are recently diagnosed with stage 1 hypertension in the office, as many as 33% may have white coat hypertension. The incidence of white coat hypertension is much lower in patients with more severe elevations of blood pressure (Am J Hypertens 1995;8:790).

Crs: A number of studies have demonstrated that patients with white coat hypertension have the same cardiovascular outcomes as normotensive patients (J Hypertens 2007;25:2193). On the other hand patients with white coat hypertension have an increased risk to develop sustained hypertension (Blood Press Monit 2000;5:249).

Lab: Daytime ambulatory blood pressure monitoring is the best way to diagnose white coat hypertension (Hypertension 2003;42:1206). In patients with white coat hypertension, the daytime blood pressures will average less than 130/85 mm Hg. Self-reported home blood pressure measurements are also valuable but are not as sensitive to detect sustained hypertension.

Rx: No treatment is advised for patients with white coat hypertension who have no evidence of target organ damage. Because there is an increased risk to develop sustained hypertension, ongoing blood pressure monitoring and assessment for target organ damage is advised.

10.5 Masked Hypertension

(Hypertens Res 2007;30:479)

Cause: Masked hypertension is when the office blood pressure is normal, but the blood pressure is elevated outside the office. Masked hypertension most commonly refers to patients who have never been diagnosed with hypertension. The criteria to define hypertension in these patients is an elevated ambulatory blood pressure greater than 135/85 mmHg. Masked hypertension can also refer to patients who are under treatment for hypertension who appear to be controlled by office blood pressure readings but are inadequately treated according to ambulatory measurements.

Epidem: The exact prevalence of masked hypertension in the population at large is unknown. The Ohasama study, conducted on a small Japanese island, found 10% of the population had ambulatory blood pressures above 133/78 mg Hg, and 3.2% were greater than 145/85 (Hypertens Res 1996;19:207). In the Pressioni Arteriose Monitorate e Loro Associazioni (PAMELA) study, 9% of the study population was found to have ambulatory blood pressures greater than 125/79 mm Hg (Circulation 2001;104:1385). Because the investigators in both of these studies used blood pressure values lower than 135/85 mmHg to define an elevated blood pressure, the true prevalence is likely lower than 10% but higher than 3%.

The Self-Measurement of Blood Pressure at Home in the Elderly: Assessment and Follow-up (SHEAF) study found that in patients being treated for hypertension, 9.4% of the patients with normal office blood pressure had elevated ambulatory readings (JAMA 2004;291:1342), and the Japan Home vs. Office Blood Pressure Measurement Evaluation (J-HOME) study found 19% in this category (Blood Press Monit 2005;10:311).

Pathophys: Masked hypertension is likely due to factors that tend to increase the blood pressure in the ambulatory setting rather than ones that would reduce it in the office setting. Cigarette smoking and alcohol use are possible contributing factors.

Crs: A meta-analysis of several large studies concluded that cardio-vascular outcomes for patients with masked hypertension are significantly worse than those for patients who are normotensive (J Hypertens 2007;25:2193). The outcomes for these patients are similar to the ones for patients with sustained hypertension.

Lab: Masked hypertension is diagnosed with ambulatory or home blood pressure monitoring. It is unclear at present who should undergo screening since the population at risk includes all nor-motensive people. Possible populations to consider are patients with other cardiovascular risk factors such as obesity and ciga-rette smoking.

Rx: There are no studies that have addressed treating this population of patients, so it is unknown whether antihypertensive therapy is effective. Smoking cession and investigation into appropriate alcohol use could be advised for patients who have those poten-tial contributing factors.

10.6   Resistant Hypertension

(J Clin Hypertens [Greenwich] 2006;8:181)

Cause: Resistant hypertension occurs when the blood pressure is not controlled with a 3-drug regimen where one of the medications is a diuretic. It is important to distinguish true resistant hypertension from apparent resistant hypertension (see Table 10.5). Apparent resistant hypertension is commonly due to patient nonadherence to the medication regimen. Other causes of apparent resistance are inaccurate measurement of the blood pressure in the office and white coat effect where the blood pressure meets goal in the ambulatory setting.

Lab: Ambulatory blood pressure monitoring can be used to evaluate blood pressure control in patients who are suspected of having the white coat effect.

For patients who have true resistant hypertension, workup for secondary hypertension is indicated. This includes tests for renovascular disease (see section 10.9), hyperaldosteronism (see Section 10.10), and pheochromocytoma (section 10.11). Urinalysis and estimation of the GFR should be performed to screen for CKD. Evaluation of sleep apnea should be considered for patients

HYPERTENSION

Table 10.5   Causes of True Resistant Hypertension

CKD
Renal vascular disease
Hyperaldosteronism
Pheochromocytoma
Obesity
Excessive salt intake
Medications that interfere with antihypertensives (eg, NSAIDs, pseudoephedrine)
Illicit drugs
Herbal medications
Sleep apnea

---

with obesity, snoring, or daytime somnolence. Echocardiography should be performed to evaluate for target organ damage (J Clin Hypertens [Greenwich] 2007;9:7).

Rx: In many cases, resistant hypertension can be controlled. Nonadherence to the medical regimen can often be difficult to recognize. If it is suspected, patient education is a critical component to improved adherence. Other intervention strategies could include improved patient–physician communication, increased clinic hours, and uncomplicated dosing schedules. Patients with CKD often require additional diuretics to attain control. Patients with other identifiable causes should respond to the appropriate intervention. For patients with true resistant hypertension without an identifiable cause, an aldosterone antagonist is a good fourth drug (Am J Hypertens 2006;19:750).

10.7 Hypertensive Crises

(Crit Care 2003;7:374)

Cause: A *hypertensive emergency* is defined as an acute elevation of systolic and diastolic blood pressures accompanied by evidence of target organ damage. Table 10.6 lists the conditions associated with hypertensive emergencies. Although no particular blood pressure requirement is part of the definition, usually the blood pressure is greater than 180/120 mm Hg (see Table 10.6).

Table 10.6   Conditions Associated with Hypertensive Emergencies

Hypertensive encephalopathy
Intracerebral hemorrhage
Acute myocardial infarction
Left-sided CHF with pulmonary edema
Unstable angina
Dissecting aortic aneurysm
Acute kidney injury
Pre-eclampsia/Eclampsia

A *hypertensive urgency* is characterized by blood pressure greater than 180/120 mm Hg but without evidence of acute organ dysfunction. Taken together, hypertensive emergencies and urgencies are termed *hypertensive crises*.

Epidem: It is estimated that up to 1% of patients who have hypertension will have a hypertensive crisis in their lifetime. This risk is higher in blacks and males. Most patients have previously diagnosed hypertension that has not been well controlled. Nonadherence to the medication regimen and the use of illicit drugs are also risk factors for the development of a hypertensive crisis. Hypertensive crises can occur in patients with essential hypertension or hypertension due to secondary causes.

Pathophys: Hypertensive crises are characterized by activation of the renin-angiotensin system, sympathetic nervous system, and vasoconstriction. When the blood pressure reaches a critical level, it causes damage to the endothelium. Intravascular coagulation (fibrinoid necrosis) and the release of local vasoconstrictors occur. When this process occurs in the kidneys, hypoperfusion of renal tissue activates the renin-angiotensin system. Tissue ischemia also activates the sympathetic nervous system. Under the influence of these hormones, the blood pressure continues to rise and causes more vessel damage, which perpetuates the vicious cycle.

Sx: These are usually related to the associated target organ.

- Hypertensive encephalopathy
  - Headache
  - Altered mental status
  - Focal neurological findings
- Cardiac manifestations
  - Chest pain
  - Dyspnea
- Kidney injury
  - Oliguria
  - Hematuria

Si: Fundoscopic findings: papilledema, retinal hemorrhages, and exudates

Lab: CBCD, electrolytes, BUN, Cr, urinalysis, EKG

Xray: CXR, CT of the head for patients with neurologic symptoms. If there are unequal pulses or a widened mediastinum, the patient should be evaluated for a dissecting aortic aneurysm.

Rx: (J Gen Intern Med 2002;17:937)

It is important to distinguish a hypertensive emergency from a hypertensive urgency. The testing available in the emergency room along with the history and physical should provide enough information to make this distinction.

Hypertensive emergency: The patient should be managed in an intensive care setting with administration of intravenous antihypertensives. The goal is to reduce the blood pressure by no more than 25% in the first hour, then bring blood pressure to 160/100 mm Hg over the next 2 to 6 hours. Exceptions to the above rule are the management of hypertension in patients with acute ischemic stroke who do not require immediate reduction in blood pressure and in patients with dissecting aortic aneurysms who should have the systolic blood pressure lowered to < 100 mm Hg, if tolerated. The drugs available for initial treatment include nitroprusside, labetalol, fenoldopam nicardipine, and esmolol. A recent review of the literature concluded that there is no best regimen for obtaining control based on outcomes.

Hypertensive urgency: Patients with severe hypertension without evidence of acute target organ damage do not require rapid lowering of the blood pressure. Oral agents are appropriate in these patients. For patients who have an established diagnosis of hypertension, augmentation of their outpatient regimen may be necessary. If nonadherence is an issue, either reinstitution or re-evaluation of the regimen requires consideration. A prompt follow-up visit should also be arranged.

10.8   Hypertension in Pregnancy

(Obstet Gynecol 2003;102:181)

Cause: There are several presentations of hypertension in the pregnant woman. *Chronic hypertension* is classified as the diagnosis of hypertension prior to pregnancy or before the 20th week of gestation. *Gestational hypertension* appears after the 20th week of pregnancy in a patient who was known to be normotensive prior to pregnancy. Severe gestational hypertension is defined as a blood pressure greater than 160/110 mm Hg. Some with hypertension will progress to *pre-eclampsia*. In addition to hypertension, women with pre-eclampsia also have proteinuria greater than 300 mg in 24 hours and edema. Severe pre-eclampsia is defined as severe gestational hypertension associated with proteinuria or severe proteinuria (> 5 g in 24 hours) associated with hypertension. Pre-eclampsia is also classified as severe if there is any organ involvement including pulmonary edema, oliguric renal failure, thrombocytopenia, abnormal liver tests with right upper quadrant pain, or any central nervous system symptoms, including headaches, blurred vision, altered mental status, and blindness. Eclampsia is the occurrence of seizures in a patient with pre-eclampsia.

Epidem: Hypertension occurs in approximately 10% of pregnancies. Patients who develop gestational hypertension are at increased risk to develop essential hypertension later in life.

Risk factors for the development of pre-eclampsia:
- Chronic hypertension
- Pre-existing renal disease
- Obesity
- Pre-eclampsia in a previous pregnancy
- Family history of pre-eclampsia
- Diabetes mellitus
- Twin pregnancies

Pathophys: (Am J Kidney Dis 2007;49:336)

The etiology of gestational hypertension, like essential hypertension, remains unknown.

During normal pregnancy, there is a drop in the diastolic blood pressure during the second trimester. This occurs despite a considerable increase in the cardiac output due to blood volume expansion. The drop is due to a dramatic decline in vascular resistance. Factors implicated in the decline in vascular resistance include progesterone-mediated smooth muscle relaxation, prolactin- and prostacyclin-mediated resistance to angiotensin II, and increased nitric oxide release. During the third trimester, the blood pressure rises under the influence of estrogen, and this is when women who develop gestational hypertension are diagnosed.

In pre-eclampsia, the characteristics that are responsible for the decline in blood pressure are reversed. There is a decrease in nitric oxide production and an increased sensitivity to angiotensin II.

Cmplc: The maternal and fetal outcomes of gestational hypertension are related to the severity of the condition. Women who develop mild gestational hypertension after the 37th week have similar outcomes as women who have normal pregnancies. Women with severe gestational hypertension have worse outcomes.

The maternal and fetal outcomes of pre-eclampsia are related to the severity of the condition and the gestational age at onset. Mild pre-eclampsia that develops after 35 weeks of gestation has similar outcomes to normal pregnancies. Women with severe pre-eclampsia that develops after 35 weeks have increased risk of maternal and perinatal morbidities. Women who develop severe pre-eclampsia earlier in pregnancy not only have increased risk of maternal and perinatal morbidities but also have increased risk of maternal and perinatal mortality.

Lab: 24-hour urine testing should be used to confirm and quantify any dipstick positive urine samples after the 20th week of gestation. Other tests that are performed to assess the severity of pre-eclampsia include CBCD with platelet count, liver function tests, and uric acid level.

Rx: (CMAJ 1997;157:1245)

The treatment goals for managing hypertension in pregnancy are to maintain maternal and fetal health. No studies have established a blood pressure goal in these patients. In addition, very few antihypertensives have been tested for safety or efficacy during pregnancy.

Chronic hypertension: Women who have hypertension prior to pregnancy should discontinue ACEIs, ARBs, atenolol, and diuretics once they know they are pregnant. They should have baseline laboratories drawn, and their blood pressure should be closely monitored. Because of the decline in diastolic blood pressure during the second trimester, they may not require any medication until late in gestation. The threshold at which to initiate treatment is unclear. Treatment of mild hypertension will reduce the incidence of severe hypertension. Methyldopa or labetalol are the first-line medications. Severe hypertension requires prompt treatment. Labetalol and hydralazine are available for oral or intravenous iv use.

Gestational hypertension: Patients with mild gestational hypertension usually undergo careful monitoring for the development of pre-eclampsia. No studies show that antihypertensives change perinatal outcomes in this group. Patients with severe hypertension should be treated similarly to patients with severe pre-eclampsia.

Pre-eclampsia: The definitive treatment for pre-eclampsia is delivery. Mild hypertension in pre-eclampsia is usually treated expectantly. If the blood pressure rises to 150/100 mm Hg or there is evidence of organ involvement, antihypertensive therapy is initiated. IV labetalol or iv hydralazine can be used in this situation.

Postpartum management: Most women with gestational hypertension become normotensive during the first week postpartum. Pre-eclampsia takes a longer time to resolve. For women who are nursing, it's important to note that most antihypertensives can be detected in breast milk.

10.9   Renovascular Disease

(J Clin Hypertens [Greenwich] 2007;9:381)

Cause: Atherosclerotic disease of the renal arteries; fibromuscular dysplasia of the renal vascular bed

Epidem: Renovascular disease accounts for about 1% of all patients with hypertension. This makes it the most common cause of secondary hypertension. Atherosclerotic disease usually presents after age 50 and is responsible for about two-thirds of the cases. Fibromuscular dysplasia of the renal arteries typically presents with hypertension developing before age 30.

There are several clinical scenarios that suggest the presence of renovascular disease:

- New onset hypertension age < 30
- Dramatic rise in blood pressure age > 50
- Resistant hypertension
- A rise in creatinine after initiation of ACEI or ARB
- Hypertension and hypokalemia
- Hypertension and other vascular disease, including coronary artery disease and peripheral arterial disease
- Hypertension associated with recurrent episodes of pulmonary edema
- A discrepancy of kidney sizes noted by renal imaging

Pathophys: Hypoperfusion of kidney tissue occurs when the renal artery lumen is occluded by more than 70%. An ischemic kidney responds by producing renin, which leads to the production of angiotensin II and aldosterone via the renin-angiotensin system. The increased production of angiotensin II is responsible for vasoconstriction, which raises the blood pressure. Hypokalemia is a consequence of the high aldosterone levels. When the renal arteries are obstructed bilaterally, aldosterone will mediate sodium and water retention. This will expand intravascular volume, further increasing blood pressure. (This also occurs when a solitary functioning kidney has a renal artery stenosis.) When the renal artery obstruction is unilateral, the normally perfused kidney will undergo a pressure diuresis, and there will be no volume overload state.

Atherosclerotic lesions tend to occur at the ostia and proximal portions of the renal arteries. They often are an extension of plaques located on the aorta. Atherosclerotic disease of the renal arteries is associated with ischemic nephropathy (J Am Soc Nephrol 2004;15:1974). Pathologic findings of arteriolar nephrosclerosis, atheroembolic disease, interstitial fibrosis, and collapse of the glomeruli are noted in the ischemic kidney. Hypoperfusion of the renal parenchyma combined with endothelial damage due to smoking, diabetes, hypertension, and hyperlipidemia are the etiologic factors.

Lesions due to fibromuscular dysplasia are usually found in the middle and distal segment of the renal arteries.

Si: Abdominal bruit is present in less than half the cases of renovascular disease.

Crs: Atherosclerotic renal artery disease commonly leads to a decline in GFR (ischemic nephropathy), especially in the presence of other risk factors for vascular disease including diabetes mellitus, smoking, and hyperlipidemia. Fibromuscular dysplasia is very rarely accompanied by loss of kidney function.

Cmplc: Hypokalemia, flash pulmonary edema; CKD, ESRD, and atheroembolic renal disease, especially in atherosclerotic renal artery disease

Lab: A number of laboratory findings suggest renovascular disease:

- Hypokalemia
- Elevated creatinine level
- Elevated plasma renin activity
- Elevated aldosterone level
- Elevated urinary ketosteroids

Xray: Generally, imaging is required to diagnose the condition. The gold standard to diagnose the condition is a renal angiogram. Unfortunately, the procedure has several risks including dye toxicity and atheroemboli.

Noninvasive screening tests include

- Duplex Doppler ultrasound renal artery imaging
- MRA of the renal arteries
- CT angiography
- Captopril renogram

A recent prospective study found the sensitivity of the MRA around 50% and the sensitivity of CT angiography around 60% for finding lesions that occlude more than half of the lumen (Ann Intern Med 2004;141:674). This is lower than several retrospective studies where the sensitivities of these tests were found to be nearer to 90% (Ann Intern Med 2001;135:401). The use of the MRA is limited in patients with CKD because of the possible development of nephrogenic skin sclerosis in these patients when exposed to gadolinium. The CT angiogram exposes patients with CKD to a potentially nephrotoxic dye load.

Duplex Doppler renal artery imaging is a technically challenging test to perform. Its sensitivity in experienced centers is 70% to 90% for detecting lesions occluding more than 70% of the lumen (Am J Roentgenol 2007;188:798).

The captopril renogram has fallen out of favor as a screening test. It has a large number of false positives, which are due to the antihypertensive effect of captopril. In addition, it is not very accurate in patients with CKD, as it is hard to differentiate reduced blood flow from reduced GFR.

Because of the imperfect nature of the screening tests for renal artery stenosis, it can be appropriate to order renal angiography in patients with a high clinical suspicion of the disease. (Prophylaxis for radiocontrast-induced kidney injury is discussed in section 3.6.) In patients where the clinical suspicion is lower, the duplex Doppler ultrasound is a good choice for patients with compromised renal function. MRA, CTA, and duplex Doppler ultrasound are all appropriate for patients with normal renal function.

Rx: Antihypertensive treatment is indicated for patients with all forms of renovascular disease. Agents that act on the renin-angiotensin axis are often very effective for lowering blood pressure. They can be used safely as long as there is not a decline in the estimated GFR by more than 30% compared to baseline or the development of hyperkalemia. The combination of ACEI and diuretic can achieve blood pressure control in up to 90% of patients. For patients with atherosclerotic disease, modification of the other risk factors is also very important. Smoking cessation, treatment of hyperlipidemia, and glycemic control are all indicated (Nephrol Dial Transplant 2005;20:1604).

For patients with fibromuscular dysplasia, treatment of the stenosis can improve blood pressure control. Results of percutaneous transmural renal angiography (PTRA) without stenting have excellent results in this group, with cure of hypertension in approximately 40% to 50% and improvement in blood pressure control in another 40% to 50% (Mayo Clin Proc 1995;70:1041).

The goal of revascularization in patients with atherosclerotic lesions is to preserve or improve renal function. Results of recent series show that 25% to 30% of patients can improve GFR after intervention, the majority of patients have no change, and 19% to 25% experience a decline in renal function (Annu Rev Med 2001;52:421). Factors that predict a poor outcome include advanced renal insufficiency with creatinine > 3.0 mg/dL, kidney size < 8 cm, or the presence of another cause of renal dysfunction, such as diabetes (Curr Hypertens Rep 2006;8:521).

Indications that could prompt revascularization are

- Resistant hypertension
- Decline in renal function despite aggressive medical therapy
- Recurrent flash pulmonary edema

PTRA with stenting is the most common procedure. Surgical intervention is generally reserved for patients with complex lesions that are not amenable to angioplastic techniques (Ann Intern Med 2006;145:901).

10.10 Hyperaldosteronism

(Clin J Am Soc Nephrol 2006;1:1039)

Cause: Primary aldosteronism associated with hypertension: Adrenal adenoma, adrenal hyperplasia.
Secondary aldosteronism associated with hypertension: Renovascular disease, diuretic therapy.
Sleep apnea and obesity are also associated with aldosterone excess.

Epidem: Primary aldosteronism is seen in up to 20% of patients with resistant hypertension. The risk of developing hypertension increases with the serum aldosterone level in normotensive patients.

Pathophys: Aldosterone is the final component in the renin-angiotensin system. Aldosterone mediated sodium retention is felt to be responsible for the development of hypertension. Aldosterone also suppresses renin production by the kidneys.

Crs: Hypertension is probably the first manifestation of hyperaldosteronism. Hypokalemia is not always present at initial presentation.

Lab: (Nat Clin Pract Nephrol 2006;2:198)

Screening for hyperaldosteronism is indicated for patients who present with hypertension and hypokalemia and for patients with resistant hypertension. Patients who develop hypokalemia on low dose diuretic therapy can also be screened. The screening tests are the plasma renin activity and the plasma aldosterone concentration. In patients with primary aldosteronism, the plasma renin activity is usually less than 1.0 ng/ml/hr, and the plasma aldosterone concentration is greater than 15 ng/dL. Renal artery disease is suggested when both tests are elevated, and licorice ingestion or hypercortisolism is suggested when both are suppressed. Aldosterone antagonists will interfere with the tests. Most other antihypertensives can be continued during testing. ACEIs and ARBs usually elevate the plasma renin activity, so a suppressed plasma renin activity while on ACEI or ARB is consistent with primary aldosteronism.

Xray: CT scanning or MRI can demonstrate an adrenal adenoma in about 30% of cases. Other patients may have adrenal hyperplasia.

Rx: Patients with an adenoma can undergo unilateral adrenalectomy. Other patients should be treated with aldosterone antagonists such as spironolactone or eplerenone.

10.11   Pheochromocytoma

(J Clin Hypertens [Greenwich] 2002;4:62)

Cause: A pheochromocytoma is a catecholamine secreting tumor.

Epidem: Pheochromocytoma is a rare cause of hypertension (< 0.05% of hypertensives). Approximately 10% are malignant. 10% to

15% are familial. The familial cases are associated with multiple endocrine neoplasia syndromes, von Hippel-Lindau disease, neurofibromatosis type 1, and carotid body tumors.

Pathophys: The symptoms of pheochromocytoma are due to excessive circulating amounts of catecholamines. Stimulation of receptors in the heart leads to tachycardia and increased contractility. Vascular receptors respond with vasoconstriction, and skin receptors respond with the production of sweat.

Sx:

- Headache
- Tachycardia
- Palpitations
- Sweating
- Pallor
- Anxiety
- Flushing during paroxysms of hypertension

Si: Paroxysmal or sustained hypertension

Crs: Can be fatal if undiagnosed

Cmplc: Congestive heart failure, cerebrovascular disease

Lab: The combination of headaches, palpitations, and sweating in a patient with sustained or paroxysmal hypertension should prompt the biochemical workup for a pheochromocytoma. The most useful biochemical screening tests are the 24-hour urinary free metanephrine analysis and plasma levels of free metanephrines (J Clin Endocrinol Metab 2003;88:4533). Abnormal elevations of these tests are very sensitive for detecting a pheochromocytoma. Testing needs to be carried out carefully as a number of medications and medical conditions can either cause elevations in catecholamine levels or interfere with the assays (see Table 10.7).

Any clinical illness associated with major stress, including acute myocardial infarction, cerebrovascular accident, and

Table 10.7   Drugs That Can Raise Catecholamine Levels

Tricyclic antidepressants
Antipsychotics
Levodopa
Withdrawal from clonidine, beta blockers, or alcohol
Cocaine abuse
Amphetamines
Phenylpropanolamine and other decongestants
MAO inhibitors combined with diet containing tyramine

cardiovascular surgery, can also increase catecholamine levels. Acetaminophen can interfere with some plasma metanephrine assays. Labetalol and sotalol can interfere with some urinary metanephrine assays. Most other antihypertensives do not interfere with the testing.

Xray: Once the presence of a pheochromocytoma has been established with the biochemical testing, imaging is required to establish the location of the tumor. About 10% are located outside the adrenal glands, but nearly all are located within the abdominal cavity. MRI of the abdomen and pelvis is the preferred test for localizing the tumor. If biochemical testing is conclusive but the tumor cannot be located by MRI, then I-123 metaiodobenzylguanidine (MIBG) scintigraphy can be ordered. This substance accumulates in most pheochromocytomas.

Rx: Patients with a pheochromocytoma should have surgical removal of the tumor. However, they also require preoperative, intraoperative, and postoperative management of their catecholamine excess. For patients with severe preoperative hypertension, iv phentolamine (an alpha blocker) can be used to control the blood pressure. Oral alpha blocking agents, including phenoxybenzamine, prazosin, terazosin, and doxazosin, are effective in the preoperative period as well. Once alpha blockade has been established, beta blockers can be used to treat tachycardia.

Intraoperative medications to avoid include atropine and fentanyl, which can cause release of catecholamines. Phentolamine, nitroglycerin, and nitroprusside can be used for intraoperative blood pressure management.

Postoperative hypoglycemia can occur after surgery due to increased insulin secretion when the catecholamine levels fall. Frequent blood glucose monitoring and an infusion of dextrose-containing iv fluids after tumor removal is indicated.

Tumor removal does not cure hypertension in all cases; as many as 25% of patients will continue to require antihypertensive medications. Patients with malignant pheochromocytomas that cannot be completely surgically resected should be treated with alpha and beta blockers along with potential chemotherapy and radiation therapy.

10.12 Hypertension in Chronic Kidney Disease

KDOQI Clinical Practice Guidelines on Hypertension and Antihypertensive Agents in Chronic Kidney Disease (Am J Kidney Dis 2004;43:S1)

Cause: CKD is one of the most prevalent causes of secondary hypertension. CKD can also be the result of target organ damage from hypertension.

Epidem: The prevalence of hypertension in patients with GFR 60-90 ml/min/1.73 m2 in the Modification of Diet in Renal Disease (MDRD) study was approximately 65% to 75% (Am J Kidney Dis 1996;28:811). 70% of patients in the Third National Health and Nutrition Examination Survey (NHANES III) study with elevated creatinine levels had hypertension (Arch Intern Med 2001;161:1207).

Pathophys: Several characteristics of CKD are associated with increased blood pressure, including activation of the renin-angiotensin system and extracellular fluid volume overload.

Cmplc: Hypertension is associated with progressive decline in GFR, increased proteinuria, and increased cardiovascular risk.

Lab: Patients with hypertension should be screened annually for CKD with an estimated GFR measurement. Patients with CKD should be screened annually for hypertension.

Rx: The target for blood pressure treatment for patients with CKD without proteinuria is 130/80 mm Hg. Medication regimens containing 2 or more medications are usually required for control. One of the medications should be a diuretic. For patients with proteinuria, the target is 125/75 mm Hg. ACEIs or ARBs are advised for patients with proteinuria or diabetics. After starting or increasing ACEI or ARB therapy, the patient should be monitored for adverse effects, including hypotension, hyperkalemia, or a decline in GFR. ACEI or ARB therapy can usually be continued as long as GFR declines less than 30% from baseline and the serum potassium is less than 5.6 mEq/L. If the decline in GFR is greater than 30%, the clinician should consider a workup for renovascular disease. If the patient develops hyperkalemia, discontinuation of other medications that could contribute to hyperkalemia (eg, potassium sparing diuretics and NSAIDs) and institution of a low potassium diet should be considered in order to continue using the ACEI or ARB.

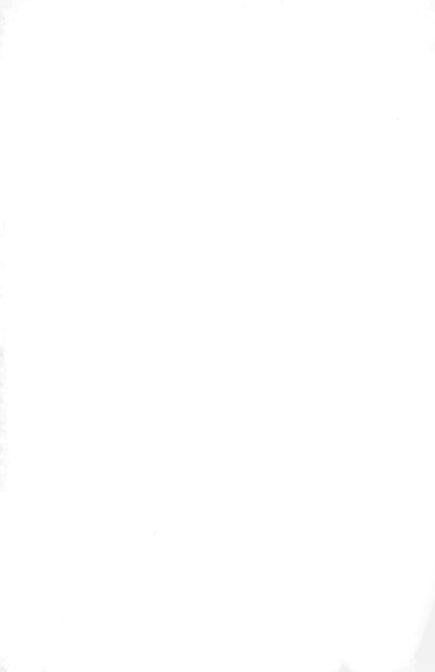

Chapter 11

Kidney Transplantation

(Arch Intern Med 2004;164:1373)

Introduction: Renal transplantation is the best treatment for ESRD for many patients. Not only does transplantation liberate the transplant recipient from the inconveniences, side effects, and other costs of dialysis, but also it allows for better survival. The difference in survival among patients who receive a transplant compared to patients fit for transplantation who remain on dialysis is dramatic. Over several years of follow-up, patients who receive a transplant experience a reduction in the risk of death of almost 70% when compared to those who are on the transplant waiting list (N Engl J Med 1999;341:1725).

In addition to the survival benefit, the outcomes of transplantation have been steadily improving for a number of years. Compared to organs transplanted in the late 1980s, organs from deceased donors transplanted in the late 1990s are estimated to last their recipients on average 3.7 yr longer with half of the kidneys still functioning after 11.6 yr. Living donor transplant recipients from the late 1990s can expect half of their transplants still to be working 19.3 yr after the transplant. That is a 6.8-yr improvement in transplant half-life compared to the late 1980s (UNOS Renal Transplant Registry 2001). Because transplantation is a better and improving therapy for ESRD, timely identification of patients fit for transplantation, and their referral to a transplant program, are critical for assuring the best outcome for this patient population.

11.1 Basic Transplant Immunology

Introduction: Improved transplantation outcomes described above are in large part due to advancements in the understanding and controlling of the antiallograft immune response. The following issues are critical in renal transplantation:

- Kidney transplantation is generally performed within the same ABO blood group compatibility context as transfusion medicine.
  - ABO blood group antigens are found on the vascular endothelial cells of the graft as well as on blood cells.
  - Antibodies to blood group antigens are present in the plasma without prior exposure.
  - These antibodies will cause intractable hyperacute rejection when an ABO incompatible organ is transplanted; thus individuals with blood group O who have preformed antibodies against A and B antigens can only have blood group O donors.
  - Blood groups O and A are most common in the United States where B is rare. Blood group B is much more common in eastern Europe and Asia. AB is rare everywhere. Individuals with blood group AB can receive a kidney from any blood group donor while people with blood group A can receive a kidney from an individual with blood group A or O.
  - A minority of individuals with blood group A have a subtype of blood group A called A2. Transplantation across the ABO rules may sometimes be possible in these individuals (Transplantation 2004;78:635).
- T Lymphocytes are critical to the kidney transplant rejection (see Figure 11.1).

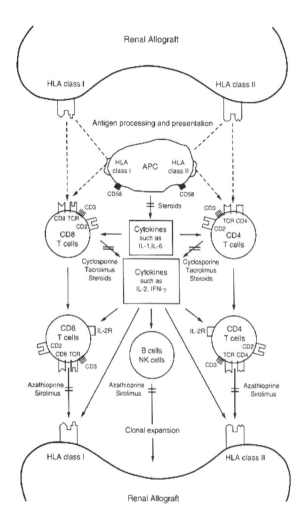

Figure 11.1 Mechanism of Anti-Allograft Response. Reprinted with permission from (N Eng S Med 1994; 331:365).

- Each T cell clone has its own unique T cell receptor.
  - A T cell receptor has similarities to the antibody in that it is clonally produced and has a variable region that is capable of recognizing fragments of specific proteins but only when they are presented on the MHC proteins, also called HLA.
  - T cells probably also recognize the HLA molecule itself, but the nature of the "transplant antigen" is incompletely understood.
  - There are 2 types of HLA that are produced by different MHC genes: class I HLA is present on all cells; class II HLA is usually present on antigen-presenting cells like macrophages but can be induced by cytokines to appear on endothelial and other cells.
  - CD8 positive T lymphocytes recognize and kill antigen-presenting cells with class I HLA and a foreign protein.
  - CD4 positive T lymphocytes do not kill antigen-presenting cells directly. They produce cytokines, particularly IL-2, which amplify the T cell response and help bring in the B cells for the initiation of antibody response.
- CD 3 complex is associated with the T cell receptor and participates in the transduction of signal into the T cell that leads to its action.
- Co-stimulation is another process that must occur simultaneously with the T cell receptor-MHC interaction to ensure T cell activation. Costimulation occurs through a different receptor family. Without co-stimulation T cells become paralyzed.
- Once T cell activation occurs, cell proliferation produces a variety of cells that attack the allograft.
- The variety of HLA proteins is possible due to polymorphism of the MHC genes. This should allow for a better immune response to a new pathogen by some subjects and should theoretically allow some people to survive any pandemic.

- Class I HLA proteins are further subdivided into types A, B, and C.
- Class II HLA proteins are further subdivided into types DP, DQ, DM, and DR.
- The 3 HLA proteins important in transplantation are A, B, and DR.
- Each person has 2 copies of each of these types of HLA, which make up the commonly discussed 6 antigens that may be matched or mismatched in kidney transplantation.
- A haplotype is the 3 HLA antigens that an individual inherited from one of his parents.
- Two siblings have a 25% chance of having a 2-haplotype match or 2-haplotype mismatch and a 50% chance of a 1-haplotype match.
- Matching all of the HLA proteins appears to confer an advantage for long-term graft survival in both living and diseased donors (N Engl J Med 2000;343:1078). The implications of various degrees of mismatch are more controversial.

11.2 Kidney Transplant Process

Introduction: Organ transplantation is a highly organized form of medical care carried out in specialized centers. A series of coordinated steps are required for a consistently successful outcome. The following steps are normally involved:

1. Referral to the transplant center
   a. Patients with progressive kidney disease can be evaluated for consideration of a preemptive transplant. (Preemptive kidney transplant is a transplant performed prior to initiation of dialysis and requires the availability of a suitable living donor.)
   b. Patients already on dialysis should be referred for consideration of transplantation if they do not have absolute

contraindications. (See evaluation of a transplant recipient below.)

2. Evaluation of the potential kidney transplant candidate (see section 11.3 for more detailed discussion of kidney transplant candidate evaluation)
   a. History and physical
   b. Consideration of the original diagnosis that led to renal failure and discussion of the risk of the recurrence of the original disease in the allograft
   c. Psychological evaluation
   d. Cancer screening
   e. Routine testing for a variety of infectious diseases
   f. Evaluation and testing for high risk conditions, such as coronary artery disease, based on history

   At this stage, many patients will be found to be poor candidates for transplantation because of high-risk conditions and will not be offered a transplant.

3. Immunologic testing
   a. ABO blood group antigens (other blood antigens such as rhesus do not affect tissue histocompatibility).
   b. HLA Antigens A, B, and DR. Since zero-mismatch transplantation is known to result in a better outcome, this information can later be used for matching the recipient to the best donor.
   c. Panel Reactive Antibodies (PRA): (Clin J Am Soc Nephrol 2006;1:404)
      Individuals who have had a previous transplant or blood transfusions or have been pregnant have had a chance to develop anti-HLA IgG antibodies that may lead to hyperacute rejection. These antibodies will be detected when the crossmatch is performed. In order to identify a patient who has a lot of preformed anti-HLA antibodies and therefore will have difficulties in having a suitable donor with

a negative crossmatch, the PRA is performed initially and then at regular intervals while the recipient remains on the transplant waiting list.

PRA is performed by adding lymphocytes from a group of individuals who are likely to be similar to local organ donors to the serum of the transplant candidate. Complement capable of attacking cells is added as well. The presence of cytotoxicity will indicate the presence of preformed anti-HLA antibodies. The results of the PRA are expressed as a percentage of the donor cells killed by the recipient's serum with complement. By knowing the HLA types of lymphocyte donors, it may be possible to determine the antigen specificities of the antibodies. A more sensitive flow cytometry PRA methodology is also available.

In its essence, PRA is an array of lymphocyte transplants into the donor serum. If the majority of these test-transplants result in failure (PRA > 50%), the potential transplant recipient is referred to as "highly sensitized." Many highly sensitized transplant candidates have preformed antibodies against most HLA and will have a great deal of difficulty finding a crossmatch negative kidney. These individuals may be able to have a transplant from an HLA identical donor, but in the absence of an HLA identical sibling, an HLA identical organ is rarely available.

At this stage, suitable candidates can be added to the national transplant waiting list or prepared for transplantation if a living donor is available.

4. Individuals with ESRD are encouraged to discuss their need for an organ and the advantages of living donor transplant with family members and appropriate nonrelatives. Potential donors can volunteer to donate a kidney. Kidney donors undergo careful screening in order to verify that they will not

be harmed by donation. (See evaluation of a potential living kidney donor below.)

5. If the donor and the recipient are ABO compatible then a crossmatch is performed.

6. Crossmatch: This test is similar to the PRA described above. Donor lymphocytes are added to the recipient's serum in the presence of complement. If the recipient has preformed IgG antibodies to the donor, HLA cell lysis will occur, and the crossmatch will be deemed positive. In most cases a positive crossmatch is an absolute contraindication for transplantation since none of the currently available immunosuppressive therapies can prevent an immediate attack on the graft by the preformed donor antibodies.

At this stage, the living donor and recipient pair can proceed to surgery. When a diseased kidney donor becomes available, his HLA profile is compared to the national database in order to allow for the optimum assignment of the zero-mismatch organs. In the United States, 17% of diseased donor transplants are from a zero-mismatch donor. If a recipient of a zero-mismatch transplant is not available, the organ is offered to an individual at the top of the transplant list in accordance with established protocols. A negative crossmatch is required for the deceased donor transplantation just like for living donor transplantation.

7. Transplant surgery
   a. Immunosuppressive therapy is initiated prior to transplantation in living donor transplant recipients and at the time of surgery in diseased donor transplant recipients.
   b. Laparoscopic donor nephrectomy is now widely offered and the possibility of faster recovery has attracted a number of donors who are interested in a less invasive surgery. Left kidney is preferred because the left renal vein is longer.
   c. The transplant kidney in adult transplant recipients is usually placed in the iliac fossa. The artery and vein are then

anastomosed to the iliac vessels. The ureter is then connected to the bladder (ureteroneocystostomy). A ureteral stent may be placed, and an antireflux tunnel is created over the ureter. Multiple renal arteries and veins may present additional challenges to the surgeon.

    d. Different surgical techniques are used in children.

8. Immediate post-transplant care may include induction immunosuppression and establishment of maintenance immunosuppression and adjustments to therapy of chronic conditions such as diabetes and hypertension. If the graft functions promptly, the hospital stay after transplant may be as short as several days.

11.3 Evaluation of Potential Kidney Transplant Candidate

(J Am Soc Nephrol 1995;6:1)

Introduction: While kidney transplantation will ultimately improve the quality and length of the recipient's life, the availability of dialysis allows time for careful preparation for transplantation with the intent of ensuring that the patient will enjoy a better quality of life and better survival than he would on dialysis. Pretransplant evaluation should include the following considerations:

- Timing of evaluation
  - Preemptive transplant (transplantation prior to needing dialysis) should be considered for all appropriate patients with CKD. This requires slowly progressive CKD, the availability of a living donor, and perfect timing.
  - Suitable candidates should be evaluated before or soon after the initiation of dialysis.

- Complete history and physical is the first step in the evaluation process. Certain areas of history deserve special attention during a transplant evaluation.
  - History of events that can lead to immunological sensitization such as blood transfusions, pregnancies, and prior transplants.
  - Availability of potential living donors, particularly of a sibling who has a 25% chance of being haploidentical.
  - History of cancer
  - Active infections
  - History of heart and vascular disease
  - Ability to participate effectively in one's medical care after transplantation
  - Active substance abuse is an absolute contraindication to transplantation.
  - Some psychiatric conditions may be a contraindication for transplantation, and a psychiatric evaluation may be appropriate.
  - Medication lists should be reviewed with attention to drugs that may be problematic after transplantation. Anticonvulsants, particularly phenobarbital, can make it difficult to achieve therapeutic levels of calcineurin inhibitors.
  - History of bladder disease, such as chronic infection or inability to empty the bladder, that is likely to be a problem after transplantation.
- Screening for infection
  - With several exceptions (hepatitis C, hepatitis B, HIV, CMV), active infection is a contraindication for transplantation. Bacterial infection should be excluded with history, physical, and routine testing for the above listed viral infections, TB and common infections such as diabetic foot problems, UTIs, dialysis access infections, peritonitis on peritoneal dialysis, and dental infections.

- Patients with hepatitis B and C, as well as HIV-positive individuals, should undergo a thorough evaluation of their condition and be placed on the optimal rx for it prior to transplantation. Cirrhosis of the liver is a contraindication for kidney transplantation. Liver biopsy may be required.
- Screening for the following infections should be undertaken prior to transplantation (Semin Nephrol 2007;27:445):
  - CMV
  - HSV
  - Hepatitis B and C
  - HIV
  - Varicella zoster virus
  - EBV
  - Syphilis
  - TB
  - Parasitic infections such as leishmania, *Cryptococcus*, strongyloides and Schistosomiasis should be excluded in endemic areas
- Patients with cholecystitis and diabetics with cholelithiasis should undergo a cholecystectomy prior to transplantation.
- Vaccinations with hepatitis A, hepatitis B vaccines and pneumococcal vaccine are recommended for individuals considered for transplantation.
- Discussion of recurrent disease risk
  - The original diagnosis that led to ESRD and the risk of recurrent disease should be discussed.
    - Hereditary nephritis, polycystic kidney disease, and reflux nephropathy cannot recur in the allograft, but other kidney diseases can, and the risk of recurrence must be discussed carefully with the patient as it may influence the decision regarding transplantation or retransplantation.
    - Less than 5% of graft loss is attributable to recurrent disease. Primary FSGS is most likely to recur in the allograft. Recurrent IgA nephropathy has a variable course and

often a good prognosis with a graft loss rate of less than 10% due to recurrent disease.

- The recurrence of diabetic nephropathy is preventable, and the ability of the patient to do all that is necessary to control diabetes should be addressed to the best extent possible, including an endocrinology consultation if required.
- Patients with hereditary nephritis have a small risk of antiglomerular basement membrane disease after transplantation, which should be discussed.

- Hypercoagulable states, such as activated protein C resistance (factor V Leiden), protein C and protein S deficiencies, and antiphospholipid antibodies, are risk factors for allograft thrombosis and early allograft loss. Transplant candidates in general and those with history of thrombosis and miscarriage in particular should be screened for hypercoagulable states. The risks and benefits of postoperative anticoagulation should be weighed on an individual basis (Am J Transplant 2002;2:872).
- Patients with severe COPD, severe pulmonary hypertension, uncontrolled asthma, and those on home oxygen should not be offered transplantation due to the high risk of death post transplant due to pulmonary disease.
- Screening for heart disease is mandatory prior to transplantation due to the high risk of death due to heart disease after the transplant. For this reason, screening for CAD and left ventricular dysfunction, both of which are common, is required. Nuclear stress testing or stress echocardiography may be appropriate for low-risk candidates. High-risk candidates should undergo coronary angiography. Due to the risk of contrast-induced nephropathy, preemptive transplant may not be possible for some patients, as they will have to wait to initiate dialysis in order to be able to have coronary angiography safely. If significant coronary artery disease (CAD) is discovered, transplantation should be delayed until it has been treated.

- The severity of cerebrovascular and peripheral vascular disease should be evaluated in patients with history of stroke or transient ischemic attack and claudication. Adequate steps must be taken to control the risk of recurrent cerebrovascular events. Some patients may require carotid endarterectomy prior to transplantation.
- Obesity confers additional risks on the transplant recipient. Individual transplant programs may develop policies regarding transplantation in obese subjects. Obesity increases a variety of risks, with wound infection being a particular concern.
- Uncontrolled secondary hyperparathyroidism and renal bone disease are likely to continue to be problems following transplantation. Subjects who are unable to achieve control of PTH with phosphorous binders, vitamin D analogs, and cinacalcet should consider having a parathyroidectomy while still on dialysis, when they can be treated with high calcium dialysate and close monitoring of laboratory parameters as part of dialysis care.
- Evaluation of bladder function may be required for patients with diabetic neuropathy
- Active cancer is a contraindication to transplantation. Patients should undergo age appropriate cancer screening, including the measurement of the prostate specific antigen as part of transplant evaluation.
  - Those with cancer in remission are usually asked to remain on dialysis for a mandatory waiting period of at least 2 yr for most cancers and as long as 5 yr for malignant melanoma and some cases of colon and breast cancer. Screening for recurrence is conducted during this period.
  - Individuals with strong family histories of colon cancer may have to undergo colonoscopy even before the recommended age prior to transplantation.
  - Transplantation is not routinely performed in patients with multiple myeloma due to multiple unacceptable risks.

- Carcinomas in situ of the bladder and cervix have a very low risk of recurrence, and a waiting period is generally not required.
- Skin cancer
  - True malignant melanoma requires a 5-yr waiting period.
  - Squamous cell carcinoma may recur and metastasize, and a 2-yr waiting period is generally required.
  - Basal cell carcinoma does not generally metastasize, and no waiting is generally required.

11.4 Evaluation of Potential Living Kidney Transplant Donor

(J Am Soc Nephrol 1996;7:2288)

Introduction: Living donor organ donation naturally brings up complex ethical issues. Not doing harm to the living kidney donor is an absolutely critical consideration in living organ donation. Individuals who are able to survive on dialysis are exposed to a great deal of physical and emotional suffering that places considerable psychological burdens on them, their families, and caregivers. It is very important to evaluate the risk to the donor separately from considering the burden of suffering by the potential recipient. It may be best to assign the living donor evaluations to a physician who is not familiar with the potential recipient's case.

The following steps are usually involved in the evaluation of the living kidney donors:

- Usually ABO typing is done first. If the donor and the recipient are not ABO compatible, no further workup is necessary. Sometimes crossmatch is done at the same time as ABO typing. Positive crossmatch can also rule out a possible living donor.
- Living donor kidney donation used to be done almost exclusively by close relatives, as it was relatively easy to be sure

of the volunteerism as the only clear motive. With expanding numbers of transplants from unrelated donors, altruistic motives may require verification that may include a formal psychological evaluation.

- Donors should be informed about the risks of nephrectomy and loss of renal reserve. In general, the rates of development of kidney disease are somewhat less in healthy kidney donors than they are in the general population. A number of cases of ESRD have been reported in kidney donors, and anyone considering kidney donation should be informed of this very small but real risk.

- Donors should be informed about inconvenient aspects of the required testing.

- Donors should be informed of financial risks related to inability to work during and after donation, as living donors are not compensated for lost wages in the United States.

- Donors should also be informed about the numerous benefits to the recipient that may include shorter time on dialysis or avoidance of dialysis altogether, better potential survival, better rehabilitation potential, and improved quality of life.

- Donors should be informed that while recipients of living donors experience 1-yr graft survival rates of well in excess of 90%, a few transplants will be lost early.

- If the risks are generally acceptable to the ABO compatible, crossmatch negative volunteer donor, the medical evaluation should be undertaken.

- Medical evaluation should begin with the review of the medical history, including medical records. The presence of CKD, proteinuria, hematuria, kidney stone disease, diabetes, hypertension, or any other chronic condition with substantial long-term risk to general health should immediately rule out a potential donor.

- Hypertension should be ruled out with multiple measurements.

- Cancer in remission at the time of donation is a special concern as it can be transmitted to the recipient in the organ.
- Infections such as HIV and viral hepatitis should be ruled out, and the CMV status of the donor should be determined. Recipients of organs from CMV positive donors will require special prophylaxis (discussed below).
- The effect of donor age on graft survival is controversial. Some series did observe inferior graft survivals with older donors while others have not. This should be carefully assessed on an individual basis.
- Kidney donors should have normal kidney function. Traditionally, 2 separate 24-hr urine collections for creatinine clearance have been used to verify normal kidney function. It may be reasonable to measure the urea clearance and calculate the estimated GFR.
- Family members of patients with PKD are at risk of having this condition themselves. It is now well established that in individuals over the age of 30 the complete absence of cysts on renal ultrasound sufficiently rules out PKD.
- Finally, a CTA is performed to ascertain that the vascular anatomy will be conducive to a good surgical outcome. One renal artery and one renal vein are most desirable. CT will also help rule out tumors and stones in the organ that is to be transplanted.
- If the above workup reveals no contraindications, the donor and the recipient may proceed to surgery.

11.5   Surgical Complications of Kidney Transplant Surgery

Introduction: A detailed description of surgical complications is beyond the scope of this book; the following is a brief description of common postoperative problems.

Renal Artery and Vein Thrombosis

(Transplant Proc 2007;39:1120)

Cause: Thrombosis can occur due to severe rejection, technical issues related to vascular anastomosis, and hypercoagulable states.

Epidem: The incidence of this complication is declining with improvements in surgical technique and better screening for hypercoagulable states.

Sx/Si: Sudden cessation of urine output in cases of arterial thrombosis and possibly hematuria and pain in cases of renal vein thrombosis

Crs: This often leads to immediate graft loss. Surgical salvage is possible only in very rare cases. Salvage is more likely with renal vein thrombosis.

Lab: Hematuria can be seen in renal vein thrombosis.

Xray: Nuclear perfusion scan will demonstrate lack of perfusion of the allograft in the event of arterial thrombosis. Duplex ultrasound can be used to evaluate venous and arterial patency.

Rx: Allograft nephrectomy when salvage is not possible.

Lymphocele

(Clin Transplant 2001;15:375)

Cause: Leakage of lymph from the disrupted lymphatics in the allograft and the patient's native lymphatic channels that travel along with the iliac vessels

Epidem: This is a relatively common complication with an incidence of approximately 20%.

Pathophys: Leakage of lymph draining from the allograft and the patient's lower extremity

Sx/Si: Pain can be present from compression of surrounding tissues. If the lymphocele compresses the iliac vein, leg edema will develop. If the lymphocele compresses and obstructs the ureter, allograft dysfunction due to obstruction will occur.

Crs: If the lymphocele is symptomatic or is causing obstruction of the ureter, spontaneous recovery is unlikely, and drainage will be required.

Cmplc: Infection of the collection

Lab: When the nature of the collection is in doubt, fluid can be aspirated under ultrasound guidance and sent for creatinine measurement and culture if infection is suspected. Lymphatic fluid creatinine should be similar to that of the serum. Urine creatinine is typically high (50–100 mg/dL), so if this level of creatinine is found in a collection, the collection is an urinoma due to a urine leak.

Xray: Ultrasound is the best modality for the evaluation of a lymphocele.

Rx: While percutaneous drainage of lymphoceles is easy to accomplish, it does not lead to resolution in most cases. Laparoscopic or open drainage of the lymphocele into the peritoneal space is the procedure of choice for the management of this complication.

Urine Leak and Ureteral Stricture

(Am J Transplant 2007;7:1536)

Cause: Urine leaks usually occur early after transplantation at the site of the connection of the transplant ureter to the bladder. Urine stricture is common in the same location, but it usually occurs much later.

Epidem: Both of these complications are rare and are seen in less than 3% of transplant recipients.

Pathophys: Urine leaks occurring at the connection of the ureter to the bladder can occur due to elevated pressure in the bladder if a Foley catheter is not in place. The distal ureter can become ischemic after being disconnected from the blood supply it was receiving from the direction of the donor bladder. Necrosis of the distal ureter will also cause a urine leak.

Sx/Si: Urine leak presents with pain due to irritation of the surrounding tissues by urine. Reduced urine output with increased output via drains or the wound may be present. Strictures of the distal ureter usually present with allograft dysfunction due to obstruction.

Lab: Elevated serum creatinine may be seen with urine leak, but renal failure may not necessarily present. Creatinine may be reabsorbed from the urine collection in the abdomen and continuously recirculated through the functioning kidney transplant. If a surgical drain is draining a urine leak, creatinine in the drainage fluid will be high.

    True findings consistent with renal failure will be present when obstructive uropathy is present due to ureteral stricture.

Xray: Nuclear medicine renal scan will demonstrate extravasation of the urine marked with the radiopharmaceutical into the abdomen.

    Urine stricture causing obstruction will cause hydronephrosis.

Rx: Placement of a ureteral stent at the time of transplant surgery followed by decompression of the bladder for several days should prevent most early urine leaks. Urine leaks due to necrosis of the distal ureter can be repaired by re-implantation of the shortened ureter into the bladder or by attaching the recipient's ureter to the donor kidney.

    Strictures of the distal ureter causing acute renal failure can be treated with a percutaneous nephrostomy. Placements of stents into the transplant ureter can be difficult via cystoscopy due to the location of the transplant ureter orifice. While the stricture can be treated with balloon dilatation, the rate of recurrence is high, and resection of the stenotic segment is the definitive therapy.

11.6 Prevention of Kidney Transplant Rejection

Introduction: The general principle of immunosuppressive therapy for rejection prophylaxis is that the immune response to the allograft tends to be most intense in the first few weeks following transplantation. All immunosuppressive protocols use more intensive immunosuppressant in the beginning followed by a gradual reduction to maintenance levels. Protocols used by different centers vary considerably. Often different approaches are used in deceased donor transplants than in living donor transplants. Especially intensive immunosuppression used in the early post-transplant period is referred to as *induction immunosuppression*. This can be accomplished by either using much larger doses of the same medications that will eventually be used for maintenance or by using specialized agents.

Specialized Agents Used for Induction Immunosuppression and Treatment of Acute Rejection

(Urol Clin North Am 2001;28:733)

Rabbit Antithymocyte Globulin: Antithymocyte globulin is manufactured by immunizing rabbits with human lymphocytes and then isolating the resulting antibodies. While the goal of using this product is to inactivate T lymphocytes, a variety of immune cells are actually affected. This agent is used for induction immunosuppression and for the treatment of rejection. Antithymocyte globulin is particularly useful in the setting of delayed graft function when maximum immunosuppression needed in the first weeks after transplant is accomplished without the use of nephrotoxic calcineurin inhibitors. This preparation can also be used for the reversal of steroid resistant acute rejection. Common adverse effects include leucopenia and thrombocytopenia. While cytokine release syndrome may occur with the first dose, it is generally milder than that seen with OKT3. The disadvantage of using this product is the increased incidence of malignancy, such as PTLD, and CMV infection when CMV prophylaxis is not used.

Anti-CD3 Monoclonal Antibody (OKT3): OKT3 is a murine monoclonal IgG antibody against the CD3 receptor. This product can be used for induction immunosuppression and reversal of acute rejection. While this preparation is highly specific for the T lymphocytes, it is seeing limited use due to the severe first dose syndrome, which occurs due to the activation of lymphocytes prior to the loss of the CD3 receptor and T cell depletion. This syndrome involves fever, hypotension, pulmonary edema, and other manifestations that make the use of this drug difficult. This drug increases the incidence of infection and PTLD in a manner similar to other T cell depleting agents. An additional problem presented by OKT3 is that its repeated use may be prevented by the development of HAMA, which may make OKT3 ineffective during subsequent use. A humanized form of OKT3 has been developed to avoid the development of HAMA.

Anti-IL2 Receptor Antibodies: Two humanized monoclonal antibodies against the IL-2 receptor, daclizumab (Zenapax) and basiliximab (Simulect), are available. When used for induction immunosuppression, these agents reduce the number and severity of acute rejection episodes. Daclizumab and basiliximab have not been demonstrated to reverse acute rejection.

Glucocorticoids: High dose glucocorticoids are frequently used for induction immunosuppression and treatment of acute rejection. Doses of methylprednisolone in the range of 500 to 1000 mg are typically used for induction of immunosuppression at the time of transplant. Much smaller daily doses are used for daily immunosuppression.

Glucocorticoids bind to a cytoplasmic receptor and are then transported into the nucleus where they induce and suppress transcription of multiple genes that, in turn, lead to a complex sequence that alters cytokine release, cell activity, and cell apoptosis.

Agents used for Maintenance Immunosuppression

(Am J Kidney Dis 2001;38:S25)

Glucocorticoids: Immediately after induction with high dose steroids, patients are placed on moderate doses of glucocorticoids such as 30 mg–60 mg of prednisone daily. These are gradually tapered to 5 to 10 mg/d, which is then continued for the life of the transplant.

Some seizure medications (phenytoin, carbamazepine, and phenobarbital) as well as rifampin decrease glucocorticoid effectiveness by inducing its metabolism. Patients treated with female sex hormones and ketoconazole will experience increased steroid effects. The adverse effects of glucocorticoids are well known and include:

- Cushingoid appearance
- Diabetes
- Hypertension
- Osteoporosis
- Avascular necrosis of the femoral head
- Cataracts
- Psychiatric problems
- Acne

Due to interest in minimizing these side effects, studies of prednisone withdrawal have been conducted and demonstrated an increased risk of graft loss (J Am Soc Nephrol 2000;11:1910).

Calcineurin Inhibitors: Cyclosporine and Tacrolimus: Although cyclosporine (Neoral and others) is a cyclic peptide consisting of 11 amino acids and tacrolimus (Progaf) is a macrolide antibiotic, they have a similar mechanism of action, which is inhibition of calcineurin, that in turn participates in the rate limiting step in T cell activation.

When cyclosporine initially became available under the trade name Sandimmune, it was often inconsistently absorbed. Subsequently, a new microemulsion formulation (Neoral) was developed. Neoral is more consistently absorbed than Sandimmune, and it also shows less blood level variability between individuals. Currently, several generic preparations considered to be bioequivalent but not identical to Neoral are available. These generic forms are not microemulsions, and thus careful monitoring of blood levels is required when patients switch from one brand of cyclosporine to another for cost reasons.

Cyclosporine preparations are usually administered every 12 hr and the whole blood trough cyclosporine level is typically measured right before the next dose. The target whole blood levels are typically 250–400 ng/ml in the early post-transplant period and 100–250 ng/ml for long-term use. Nephrotoxicity is one of the principal side effects of concern in renal transplantation, and therefore careful monitoring of drug levels is necessary. It has been suggested that measurement of cyclosporine levels 2 hr after dose administration might better predict the overall cyclosporine exposure; however, this method is yet to be proven and fully accepted (Transplantation 2007;83:1525). IV formulation of cyclosporine is available for patients who are unable to take drugs by mouth. IV cyclosporine is administered by a long infusion at one-third of the daily oral dose.

Detailed knowledge of calcineurin inhibitor drug interactions is necessary for the care of transplant recipient. Interactions with some of the commonly used drugs are shown in Table 11.1. Cyclosporine can lead to accumulation of HMG-CoA inhibitors used for the treatment of hyperlipidemia. This can lead to an increased risk of myopathy and rhabdomyolysis as well as abnormal liver function tests.

Table 11.1 Calcineurin Inhibitor and Sirolimus Drug Interactions

Increases Calcineurin Inhibitor Levels	Decrease Calcineurin Inhibitor Levels
Antihypertensives	Anticonvulsants
Diltiazem	Phenobarbital
Verapamil	Phenytoin
Antibiotics	Carbamazepine
Antibacterial	Antibiotics
Erythromycin	Anti-tuberculosis medications
Clarithromycin	Rifampin
Antifungals	Isoniazid
Ketoconazole	Antibacterial
Fluconazole	Ciprofloxacin
Itraconazole	Trimethoprim/Sulfamethoxazole
Anti-HIV	Psychiatric
Protease Inhibitors	Nefazodone
Indinavir, ritonavir, saquinovir, nelfinavir	Herbal remedies
Immunosupressants	St John's Wort
Sirolimus (Increases Cyclosporine level)	
Methylprednisolone	
Grapefruit juice	

Tacrolimus is similar to cyclosporine in its mechanism of action, nephrotoxicity, and drug interactions. Target whole blood concentrations of tacrolimus are 8–15 ng/ml immediately after transplantation and 5–12 ng/ml during later periods. Tacrolimus is more effective than cyclosporine in preventing acute rejection after transplantation (Transplantation 1997;64:436), but it does not improve 1-yr graft survival. Tacrolimus was also demonstrated to be effective in reversal of refractory acute rejection episodes (Transplantation 1996;62:594). This has led some transplant programs to use tacrolimus as the first line calcineurin inhibitor for all patients immediately after transplantation, while other programs have reserved it for individuals at high immunological risk or for those with history of acute rejection. Even though tacrolimus is more effective at preventing acute rejection, concern about the increased risk of developing PTDM continues to makes the use of cyclosporine as the first-line drug attractive in nondiabetics. Newer approaches, which combine lower dose tacrolimus with MMF and induction therapy, may prove advantageous, but long-term data is not yet available (N Engl J Med 2007;357:2562).

Some side effects are more likely to happen with one agent compared to the other, which may allow for individualization of treatment for many patients:

- Cyclosporine is more likely to cause hypertension than tacrolimus (78% vs 28% at 4 months); this may be an advantage given the high risk of cardiovascular complications in transplant recipients (Transplantation 1993;55:1332).
- Cyclosporine is likely to cause unfavorable changes to the patient's lipid profile, and switching from cyclosporine to tacrolimus improves the lipid profile (J Am Soc Nephrol 2001;12:368).
- PTDM probably occurs more commonly in the patients treated with tacrolimus than with cyclosporine. A number of other factors such as age, race, and intensity of steroid therapy make the assessment of the magnitude of the increased risk of PTDM with tacrolimus as compared to cyclosporine difficult. A number of excellent publications on this subject are available (Am J Kidney Dis 1999;34:1; Transplantation 2006;81:335). Some transplant programs use tacrolimus as the calcineurin inhibitor of choice for patients who are already diabetic while using cyclosporine for average immunological risk patients in order to manage the risk of new onset PTDM.

- Neurological side effects such as tremors and headaches are more common with tacrolimus.
- Cosmetic side effects such as hirsutism and gingival hyperplasia are seen more commonly with cyclosporine. These side effects may be particularly important in specific patient groups such as young women.
- Tacrolimus is the preferred agent in children, who may especially benefit from the reduction in glucocorticoid doses that may be possible with this more potent immunosuppressant.
- Hyperuricemia and gout are seen with both calcineurin inhibitors.
- Hyperkalemia and hypomagnesemia can be seen with both of these drugs.

Acute calcineurin inhibitor nephrotoxicity is due to intrarenal vasoconstriction. This will result in elevation of creatinine, which will be exacerbated by volume depletion when toxic blood levels are present. Typically, creatinine will improve as the levels come down. The chronic renal lesion of calcineurin inhibitor toxicity involves arteriolar hyalinosis and interstitial fibrosis. This lesion is seen not only in renal transplants but also in the native kidneys of non-kidney transplant recipients. Cyclosporine and tacrolimus can cause TMA. This probably occurs due to direct endothelial injury that may be limited to the renal allograft. Conversion to a noncalcineurin inhibitor-containing regimen is the best approach to calcineurin inhibitor-induced TMA.

Sirolimus: Sirolimus, also called rapamycin and marketed under the trade name Rapamune, is a newer immunosuppressive agent. Sirolimus binds to the same intracellular receptor as tacrolimus but instead of inhibiting calcineurin, sirolimus acts on the MTOR, which is an enzyme important in cytokine-induced cell proliferation. Sirolimus blocks T cell proliferation as well as proliferation of some other cells. Sirolimus is administered once daily to achieve the target level of 5–15 ng/ml. Sirolimus was originally used in combination with cyclosporine instead of aza-thioprine. Sirolimus, like calcineurin inhibitors, is metabolized by the CYP3A4. It was subsequently noted that sirolimus interferes with cyclosporine metabolism and may exacerbate cyclosporine but not tacrolimus nephrotoxicity. For this reason, sirolimus should be administered 4 hr after the dose of cyclosporine. Since sirolimus is not nephrotoxic, there is considerable interest in designing calcineurin inhibitor-free protocols that include this agent. Sirolimus has been shown to be associated with worsen-ing proteinuria in certain patient groups and caution is required when using this drug in patients with proteinuria.

Side effects of sirolimus include hyperlipidemia, anemia, and thrombocytopenia. Sirolimus can cause interstitial pneumonitis that usually occurs during the first 6 months after initiation of the drug. Because sirolimus is metabolized by the same cyto-chrome P450 pathway as calcineurin inhibitors, it will be subject to many of the same drug interactions shown in Table 11.1.

Azathioprine: Azathioprine is a purine analog that interferes with DNA synthesis and lymphocyte proliferation. Prior to the intro-duction of cyclosporine, azathioprine and prednisone were the standard therapy used in all renal transplant recipients. Aza-thioprine is inexpensive, and it is still used in combination with prednisone and cyclosporine at some transplant centers. Azathio-prine can cause anemia, leucopenia, thrombocytopenia, hepatitis, and rarely pancreatitis. Patients receiving azathioprine should be monitored for these side effects, and the drug should be reduced or discontinued when they are noted. Allopurinol, a xanthine oxidase inhibitor, interferes with degradation of some of the active metabolites of azathioprine. This may lead to a potentially devastating myelosuppression. Concomitant use of azathioprine and allopurinol should be avoided.

Mycophenolate Mofetil and Enteric-coated Mycophenolate:

MMF (CellCept) and enteric-coated **mycophenolate sodium** (Myfortic) inhibit de novo purine synthesis and lymphocyte proliferation in a manner similar to azathioprine. MMF was initially introduced in 1995. It was found to be more effective than azathioprine when used in large doses in combination with older cyclosporine preparations. Today, MMF is widely used in a number of transplant regimens. Enteric-coated mycophenolate sodium was introduced more recently in an attempt to overcome the well-known gastrointestinal side effects of MMF. It is not clear at this time that enteric-coated mycophenolate sodium is superior to MMF when it comes to gastrointestinal side effects, which are believed to be largely due to the systemic effects of mycophenolic acid.

MMF is usually prescribed at the dose of 1000 mg twice a day, although the doses of 1500 mg twice a day can be used. Enteric-coated mycophenolate sodium at 720 mg is equivalent to 1000 mg of MMF. Even though MMF is not metabolized by the cytochrome P450 system, it is believed to have an interaction with tacrolimus that increases blood levels of MMF. The dose of 2 g/d should not generally be exceeded in patients who are also on tacrolimus. Higher than usual doses of MMF may be required to achieve similar graft outcomes in African Americans for whom the dose of 3 g/d may be more appropriate (Transplantation 1997;64:1277). MMF should be used at reduced doses in combination with sirolimus, as both drugs may cause leucopenia and thrombocytopenia.

Gastrointestinal side effects are common with MMF and may include nausea, vomiting, diarrhea, and dyspepsia. Hematological side effects on any cell line may also occur and require periodic monitoring. MMF should not be used in patients who are pregnant or want to become pregnant; azathioprine is a better choice in these patients.

Infection Prophylaxis:

(N Engl J Med 1994;331:365)

Routine antimicrobial prophylaxis against the most problematic infections is widely utilized during the initial post-transplant period. Typically, routine prophylaxis includes the following:

- Trimethoprim-sulfamethoxazole is used to prevent *Pneumocystis jiroveci* (formerly *Pneumocystis carinii*) pneumonia. It also prevents urinary tract infections. This is typically continued for several months after transplantation.
- Antifungal prophylaxis for the prevention of oral candidiasis is routinely utilized in the early post-transplant period. Topical treatments such as nystatin or clotrimazole are typically used.
- CMV prophylaxis with ganciclovir is routinely utilized in CMV-negative recipients of CMV-positive kidneys and in CMV-positive recipients. The former group is at the highest risk of clinical CMV disease.

11.7   Rejection

(Am J Kidney Dis 2004;43:1116)

Introduction: Kidney transplant rejection is classified based on its severity and the underlying immunological mechanism; while some overlap between different types of rejection may exist, the classification system shown below is generally useful. With modern immunosuppressive regimens, only 10% to 20% of patients will experience acute rejection, and most of these are due to acute cellular rejection.

Hyperacute Rejection

Cause: Presence of preformed antibodies to HLA or blood group antigens

Epidem: Should be exceedingly rare when proper blood group typing and crossmatch are performed

Pathophys: Binding of the preformed antibodies to the vascular endothelium with immediate graft thrombosis

Sx/Si: Usually happens during surgery with patients still under anesthesia

Crs: Immediate graft loss due to thrombosis

Cmplc: Rupture of the graft due to thrombosis

Lab: ABO mismatch or positive crossmatch will be present and should have been detected prior to surgery.

Kidney Bx: Thrombosis and ischemic necrosis

Rx: Graft removal and return to dialysis

Acute T Cell-Mediated Rejection (Acute Cellular Rejection)

Cause: T cell response to the allograft due to inadequate immunosuppression. The differential diagnosis of inadequate immunosuppression includes the following:

- Under-dosing of medications due to desire to wean a variety of immunosuppressants for a number of possible reasons that may include ongoing complications such as infection or severe glucocorticoid side effects
- Introduction of agents that induce the metabolism of calcineurin inhibitors and sirolimus (see Table 11.1)
- Failure to dose medications according to patient characteristics, such as failure to dose azathioprine for body weight and failure to administer 3000 mg of MMF per day to individuals with large body size and to African Americans
- Medication noncompliance

Epidem: Of the 10% to 20% of patients who will experience an acute rejection episode, 90% will have acute cellular rejection of the interstitial type.

Pathophys: Infiltration of the kidney with T lymphocytes

Sx/Si: Most cases are completely asymptomatic and are detected with routine laboratory monitoring. Occasionally a tender allograft and decreased urine output may be seen.

Crs: This is usually seen in the first several weeks after transplantation. It can present as delayed graft function just days after transplantation. Occurrence of this complication late after transplant is usually due to medication noncompliance.

Cmplc: Failure to recover allograft function to the previous level or graft loss

Lab: Increase in serum creatinine. Serum creatinine should be measured frequently in the initial post-transplant period.

Kidney Bx: A kidney biopsy is the definitive intervention needed for the diagnosis of rejection. *Tubulitis* (infiltration of the tubular compartment by lymphocytes and other inflammatory cells) is the classic finding seen in acute rejection. Banff classification is used to type acute rejection episodes and to grade their severity. While tubulitis is often seen in rejection, 2 other conditions may produce this biopsy appearance:

- BK polyomavirus nephropathy
- Post-transplant lymphoproliferative disorder or lymphoma infiltrating the allograft

Rx: In general, empiric treatment of acute rejection prior to allograft biopsy requires caution. The 10% to 20% incidence of acute rejection is similar to the incidence of BK polyomavirus nephropathy at about 10%. Since empiric pulse glucocorticoids would likely worsen the course of the BK polyomavirus nephropathy, this therapy should be delayed until the diagnosis of rejection is confirmed by biopsy. Ideally, BK polyomavirus viremia and viruria should be excluded as well.

Three major approaches to the therapy of an acute rejection episode are available:

1. Pulse high dose glucocorticoids for several days is a commonly used approach. This is usually followed by intensification of baseline immunosuppression or restoration of baseline immunosuppression in cases of prior under-dosing and noncompliance. If transplant function fails to improve after 5 to 7 d, the episode is deemed steroid resistant. As many as 30% of the cases may be steroid resistant.
2. Antibody preparations such as rabbit antithymocyte globulin given for several days can be utilized. There is evidence that this approach is more effective than pulse glucocorticoids (Transplantation 2006;81:953).
3. Conversion to a rescue form of immunosuppression that may be more effective than a previous regimen is the third approach. Conversion from cyclosporine to tacrolimus, as well as substitution of MMF for azathioprine, is frequently utilized.

Antibody-Mediated (Humoral) Rejection

Cause: Antibodies against donor HLA

Epidem: This form of rejection represents about 10% of the cases of acute rejection; it may coexist with cellular rejection.

Patients who have undergone desensitization for anti-HLA antibodies and those with high PRA titers prior to transplantation are at risk of this complication.

Pathophys: Anti-HLA antibodies and possibly antibodies to other endothelial antigens mediate humoral rejection.

Sx/Si: Increase in serum creatinine is the most common presentation.

Crs: Untreated rejection will lead to graft loss. Humoral rejection with diffuse C4d staining has a poor prognosis. In one series, diffuse positive staining for C4d was associated with a 65% rate of graft loss at 1 yr, while focal staining for C4d was associated with a 33% rate of graft loss at 1 yr (Transplantation 2005;79:228).

Cmplc: Graft loss and treatment complications related to intensive immunosuppression and plasma exchange.

Lab: In addition to rising serum creatinine and urinary abnormalities, donor specific antibodies may be detectable in the recipient's blood.

Kidney Bx: Acute glomerular capillary inflammation that has the appearance of vasculitis with cellular pericapillary infiltrates, inflammation, and necrosis of vascular structures. Positive staining of peritubular capillaries for C4d is typically seen in cases of humoral rejection.

Rx: Plasma exchange and/or iv immune globulin is usually utilized to remove the preformed antibodies. Additional therapies with pulse steroids and antilymphocyte antibodies, such as OKT3, must be utilized to reduce antibody production and to prevent replacement of antibodies removed by the plasma exchange.

Chronic Allograft Nephropathy

(Semin Nephrol 2007;27:414; N Engl J Med 2003;349:2326)

Cause: Several insults can initiate the changes of CAN. The most common are ischemic injury, severe or subclinical rejection, and drug toxicity.

Epidem: Chronic allograft nephropathy is the most common cause of graft loss in living patients. Findings consistent with CAN are seen in 90% of protocol biopsies done at 1-yr post-transplant.

Pathophys: Insults described above eventually lead to vascular, glomerular, and interstitial damage in the allograft.

Sx/Si: The initial stages of CAN are asymptomatic. Patients who develop heavy proteinuria may become edematous. As allograft dysfunction progresses, sx/si of uremia will develop.

Crs: Chronic allograft nephropathy often results in progressive allograft dysfunction and graft loss.

Cmplc: Allograft loss

Lab: Proteinuria, occasional hematuria, and findings consistent with progressive renal dysfunction

Kidney Bx: The biopsy will reveal an MPGN pattern of injury. Vessels will show fibrointimal proliferation. In the interstitial compartment, progressive fibrosis and tubular atrophy will be seen. The Banff grading system grades these findings based on severity, which also helps with prognosis.

Rx: Prevention of CAN is an important consideration. Adequate immunosuppression must be provided to avoid acute rejection episodes that have a significant negative effect on prognosis. Similarly, care should be taken to avoid other insults when possible. These include infection and drug toxicity. Conversion from calcineurin inhibitors to the non-nephrotoxic sirolimus can be considered with caution. Sirolimus has been associated with increased and new proteinuria in this setting (Nephrol Dial Transplant 2005;20:2517). In addition, there is concern about increased risk of infection in patients with failing transplants after sirolimus conversion.

11.8   Infection in Kidney Transplant Recipients

(N Engl J Med 2007;357:2601; Semin Nephrol 2007;27:445)

Introduction: Transplant recipients are susceptible to a variety of infections. These patients are immunosuppressed and have impaired defenses due to dialysis access and other devices. In addition, these patients are exposed to a variety of pathogens, some of which are nosocomial. Latent donor and recipient pathogens, such as CMV, may also play a role. Management of these patients is further complicated by the fact that these infections present with mild or no symptoms and that infection with several pathogens at once is not unusual. Many infections occur during predictable time windows following transplantation due to

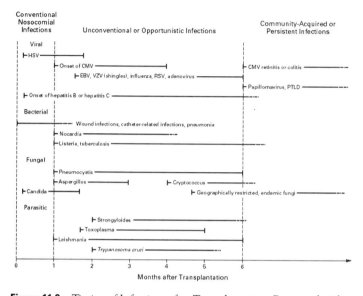

Figure 11.2 Timing of Infections after Transplantation. Reprinted with permission from (N Engl J Med 1998; 338:1741).

unique intensity and duration of immunosuppression associated with these infections as well as changing epidemiologic factors (see Figure 11.2).

While discussion of most infectious complications is beyond the scope of this book, CMV, BK polyomavirus, and PTLD are discussed in detail below.

Cytomegalovirus Infection in Renal Transplantation

(J Am Soc Nephrol 2001;12:848; Lancet 2005;365:2105)

Cause: CMV belongs to the family Herpesviridae.

Epidem: Prior to widespread introduction of routine prophylaxis, the incidence of CMV disease was between 20% and 60%. Introduction of routine prophylaxis has reduced the incidence to 5%.

The probability of disease occurrence is related to the recipient and donor status. Active infection is most likely when a CMV-negative recipient receives a CMV-positive allograft.

Pathophys: White blood cells are the reservoir for the virus. The virus infects cells through fusion of the viral envelope with the cell membrane. This virus can infect almost any tissue. The most common clinical syndromes are listed below:

- Syndrome of low-grade fever, malaise, and low wbc count
- Pneumonia
- Hepatitis and infection of the pancreas and gallbladder
- Stomach ulcerations and/or colitis
- Retinitis and CNS infection
- Myocarditis
- Kidney allograft and ureter infections (renal failure due to CMV is uncommon)

Sx/Si: Site specific

Crs: CMV disease is treatable if promptly recognized.

Cmplc: Depends on site of involvement. Severe pneumonia and colon perforation may occur.

Lab: A number of methodologies for detection of CMV are available:

- Serological studies for CMV IgG and IgM are available. A high IgM titer or a dramatic increase in the IgG titer is indicative of active infection.
- Rapid CMV culture, by the shell vial method, of the involved tissue (buffy coat of the centrifuged blood, urine, bronchoalveolar lavage, etc) can be utilized for the diagnosis of active infection at those specific sites.
- Viremia can be detected with an assay for a pp65 viral antigen or by PCR viral load assays.

Xray: Various imaging modalities are available depending on involved site.

Rx: The following prophylactic approaches can dramatically reduce the incidence of CMV disease:

- Using leucoreduced and/or CMV-negative red blood cell products for transfusion
- Using oral ganciclovir or oral valganciclovir for prophylaxis when the donor, the recipient, or both are CMV positive prior to transplantation. The duration of therapy was 100 d in one study of these agents in the highest risk patients (Am J Transplant 2004;4:611).

Active disease is treated with iv ganciclovir. For severe disease, a reduction of immunosuppression is required. CMV hyperimmune globulin can also be utilized for the treatment of severe infections. Valganciclovir has the advantage of excellent oral bioavailability; however, iv ganciclovir remains the standard of care at this time. When tissue invasive CMV infection is diagnosed, it is likely that other infections are present. This is an important consideration because multiple infections will need to be diagnosed and treated; for example, CMV and *Pneumocystis jiroveci* (formerly *Pneumocystis carinii*) pneumonias may require simultaneous therapy.

BK Polyomavirus Nephropathy

(Clin J Am Soc Nephrol 2007;2[suppl 1]:S36)

Cause: BK polyomavirus: This virus is in the same family as the JC polyomavirus that causes PML.

Epidem: Between 60% and 80% of patients have detectable antibodies against BK virus due to infection during childhood. These antibodies do not prevent reactivation and nephropathy in kidney transplant patients. Most patients who experience reactivation of the virus do not develop overt nephropathy but do have a detectable virus at least in the urine. The following percentages of patients will experience at least one manifestation of the virus:

- Viruria, 30%–40%
- Viruria and decoy cells on urine cytology, 20%–30%
- Viruria, decoy cells and viremia, 10%–20%
- Nephropathy is seen in up to 10% of patients who also usually have viruria, decoy cells, and viremia
- Nephropathy without viremia is rare

It is important to note that with modern immunosuppression the incidence of acute rejection (10%–20%) is generally similar to the rate of BK virus nephropathy causing acute allograft dysfunction (around 10%). This should lead to caution when empiric treatment of rejection is being considered.

Pathophys: BK polyomavirus, present in the body since childhood, undergoes activation and replication in kidney transplant recipients. Typically, viruria develops first, and some patients go through the above stages in order. The virus can be detected in a variety of urothelial cells. In patients with overt nephropathy, the virus causes infection and destruction of the tubular epithelial cells followed by the destruction of peritubular capillary walls. This allows the virus to enter the bloodstream and become detectable in blood. Immune response to infected tubular cells leads to tubulitis and other inflammatory responses within the graft.

Sx/Si: This disease is generally asymptomatic unless severe nephropathy leads to graft loss and uremia.

Crs: Not all patients will have a poor prognosis, especially if immunosuppression is reduced once viral replication is detected.

Cmplc: Graft loss and the failure to distinguish tubulitis due to BK virus from rejection. Increasing immunosuppression in an attempt to treat misdiagnosed rejection can lead to worsening BK virus nephropathy.

Lab: Testing for BK virus DNA in blood or urine should be undertaken whenever unexpected allograft dysfunction develops, particularly in the initial post-transplant period and whenever a biopsy is performed. In addition, an expert panel recommends screening for BK virus replication by PCR every 3 months during the first 2 yr post-transplant (Transplantation 2005;79:1277). Annual testing up to post-transplant yr 5 has also been recommended. PCR assays for BK virus DNA in blood and urine are available. The presence of more than 10,000 copies of BK virus DNA per ml of plasma or more than 1×10^7 copies per ml of urine have a positive predictive value of between 50% and 85% for the presence of biopsy proven BK virus nephropathy. Decoy cells can be detected by urine cytology. Decoy cells are shed tubular epithelial cells with viral inclusion bodies.

Kidney Bx: The presence of basophilic intranuclear inclusions will help distinguish BK virus nephropathy from tubulitis due to rejection. Tubular atrophy and fibrosis can be seen. If the inclusion bodies are not seen, BK viremia and viruria can help distinguish between acute rejection and BK virus nephropathy.

Rx: Reduction of immunosuppression is the only available treatment for BK virus nephropathy. For patients on a 3-drug regimen, discontinuation of azathioprine or MMF is generally recommended. Reduction in immunosuppression may be reasonable in any patient with viremia detected on routine screening. Reduction in viral loads will usually take several months. Patients who lose their grafts due to BK virus nephropathy can be retransplanted. In most cases, removal of the failed allograft has been performed prior to retransplantation.

Leflunomide, an agent that interferes with DNA synthesis and approved for the treatment of rheumatoid arthritis, has been used for treatment of BK virus nephropathy using a complex approach, which involved monitoring of the blood level of an active metabolite (Transplantation 2006;81:704). This approach led to decrease in the BK virus viral load and stabilization but not the improvement in renal function.

Cidofovir is an antiviral agent with activity against the BK polyomavirus. The use of this agent is limited by its nephrotoxicity.

Post-transplantation Lymphoproliferative Disorders

(Clin Chest Med 2005;26:631; Pediatr Clin North Am 2003;50:1471)

Cause: Most cases are due to EBV. Some cases are EBV negative and are poorly understood.

Epidem: PTLD is seen in about 1% of adult transplant recipients. PTLD is much more common in children in whom it has a somewhat different pathophysiology. This complication occurs most commonly during the first post-transplant year.

Pathophys: Most cases of PTLD are due to EBV-induced proliferation of B lymphocytes. Several classifications of PTLD exist. Three major groups represent the spectrum of disease (Blood 1995;85:552):

1. Benign illness clinically resembling mononucleosis. This form is seen in about half of the patients with PTLD. This condition is due to nonmalignant polyclonal B cell proliferation.
2. Polymorphic B cell hyperplasia or lymphoma is a monoclonal disorder that may be seen in the nodes or in extranodal sites.
3. Widely disseminated and often extranodal disorder with various oncogene and tumor suppressor gene mutations.

Sx/Si: Patients with benign B cell proliferation will present with fever, tonsilar enlargement, and cervical lymphadenopathy. Patients with more malignant forms of the disease will have fevers, weight loss, and palpable masses in some cases. The kidney transplant may be involved with resulting renal failure. In general, symptoms will be related to the involved site; for example, central nervous system lymphoma may present with vague neurological symptoms.

Crs: The course will depend on the type of disease. Patients with benign polyclonal disease will respond to reduction of immunosuppression. Patients with more malignant disease may have a poor prognosis. As with most malignant disorders, prognosis will depend on performance status.

Cmplc: Oncological complications related to radiation and chemotherapy

Lab: While measurement of EBV viral load is possible, the diagnosis is typically made by biopsy of the affected site.

Xray: Various imaging techniques may be utilized based on the involved site. Positron emission tomography can be used to confirm the presence of malignant tissue in a variety of body sites.

Rx: The benign polyclonal form of the disease will often respond to reduction of immunosuppression. Antiviral therapies with acyclovir and ganciclovir have been utilized in an attempt to control viral replication. Cells that have undergone malignant transformation will not respond to antiviral therapy. More severe forms of the disorder will require chemotherapy and/or radiation, and sometimes surgery, in an attempt to control the disease.

11.9 Miscellaneous Conditions of Importance during the First Post-transplant Year

Post-transplant Erythrocytosis

(Am J Kidney Dis 1994;24:1)

Cause: Poorly understood

Epidem: This complication is seen in about 15% of transplant recipients. It is seen more often in males.

Pathophys: Excessive production of erythropoietin by the native kidneys has been proposed as one possible explanation. Enhanced sensitivity to erythropoietin and possible stimulation of erythroid precursors by angiotensin II have also been implicated.

Sx/Si: None unless complications develop

Crs: Spontaneous resolution is unlikely, and elevated hemoglobin and hematocrit are likely to persist.

Cmplc: Hypertension, DVT, and stroke can occur as a result of erythrocytosis.

Lab: In order to meet the definition of this condition, hematocrit must be persistently elevated above 51%.

Xray: The differential diagnosis of elevated hematocrit post-transplant includes the possibility of an erythropoietin-secreting renal cell carcinoma of the native kidneys. This can be ruled out with CT or US.

Rx: If a hypertensive emergency or another serious complication is present, therapeutic phlebotomy may be performed. Chronically, ACEIs and angiotensin receptor blockers are utilized with good results. Low doses of ACEIs are often effective.

Persistent Post-transplant Hyperparathyroidism

(J Am Soc Nephrol 2002;13:551)

Cause: Persistence of hyperparathyroidism, which developed in the course of CKD and while on dialysis

Epidem: 50% of kidney transplant recipients still have hyperparathyroidism 1 yr after transplantation. In addition, about one-half of all transplant recipients have hypercalcemia after transplantation.

Pathophys: Secondary hyperparathyroidism of uremia that develops during the period of CKD and while individuals are on dialysis often does not resolve immediately upon transplantation. After a successful transplant, uremia, phosphorous retention, and skeletal resistance to PTH resolve, but oversecretion of PTH persists. This in turn can lead to hypercalcemia, hypophosphatemia, and bone loss. The bone loss which is at least in part due to immuno-suppressive medications leads to an increased risk of fracture.

Sx/Si: Bone pain can occur. Hypercalcemia can result in development of symptomatic kidney stones.

Crs: Depends on allograft function. Patients with good allograft function may eventually have normalization of PTH and bone metabolism.

Cmplc: Fracture, bone pain, and kidney stones

Lab: Elevated PTH, hypercalcemia, and hypophosphatemia

Xray: Bone density measurement with dual-energy Xray absorptiometry

It is important to note that the use of bone density informa-tion for predicting fracture risk after renal transplantation may not have the same utility as it does in postmenopausal osteoporo-sis. In particular, it is not clear that DEXA bone density informa-tion can be used to predict the risk of distal fractures that are common in this population.

Rx: Prevention of post-transplant hyperparathyroidism begins with maintaining PTH in the optimum range prior to transplantation. Post-transplant, the dose of glucocorticoids should be maintained at the lowest effective level to prevent bone loss. If hypercalce-mia is not present, calcium supplementation should be provided along with vitamin D. If bone density is low post-transplant or if rapid loss of bone density is occurring while allograft function is good, bisphosphonates can be used along with exercise.

11.10 Long-term Care of a Kidney Transplant Recipient

(Clin J Am Soc Nephrol 2006;1:623)

Introduction: While short-term outcomes of kidney transplantation have improved considerably, long-term outcomes in patients treated with transplantation remain less than optimal, not only due to poor allograft function but also due to substantial morbidity and mortality related to other comorbidities. Because of the substantial impact of these comorbid complications on patient outcomes, long-term follow-up of transplant recipients should include careful attention to those conditions along with care directly related to allograft function and CKD. It is important to remember that the mortality rate of kidney transplant recipients is higher than that of individuals with other forms of CKD at the same level of kidney function.

Cardiovascular Disease

Cardiovascular disease is the principal cause of mortality in kidney transplant recipients. Many transplant recipients also develop cerebrovascular and peripheral vascular disease. While routine screening for coronary artery disease is not recommended at this time, a high index of suspicion is required for those who provide routine health care for renal transplant recipients.

Hypertension

The incidence of post-transplant hypertension may be as high as 80%. A number of factors contribute to the high incidence and severity of hypertension in this population. These include abnormal kidney function, use of calcineurin inhibitors and corticosteroids, preexisting hypertension, and transplant renal artery stenosis. Hypertension should be treated aggressively in renal transplant recipients with a goal BP of less than 130/80 mm Hg with lifestyle modification and antihypertensive medications. The use of ACEIs and ARBs is appropriate and safe in renal transcript recipients in general and those with proteinuria in particular. Caution should be used during the concurrent titration of calcineurin inhibitors and ACEIs and ARBs as both can cause an increase in serum creatinine. A 30% rise in serum creatinine is expected and appropriate with ACEI and ARB therapy.

Dyslipidemia

Dyslipidemia is a risk factor for CAD, death, and graft loss. In renal transplant recipients, dyslipidemia may be exacerbated by corticosteroids and sirolimus as well as by comorbid conditions such as post-transplant diabetes. Treatment of dyslipidemia after transplant can result in substantial improvements in survival, and it is therefore recommended (Am J Kidney Dis 2002;40:638). Caution is needed when statins (HMG-CoA reductase inhibitors) are used concurrently with calcineurin inhibitors due to the significant drug interaction between these drug classes that will dramatically increase patients' statin exposure and the risk of statin toxicity, particularly rhabdomyolysis (Drugs 2003;63:367).

Post-transplant Diabetes Mellitus

(Endocrinol Metab Clin North Am 2007;36:907)
Up to 25% of renal transplant recipients will develop post-transplant diabetes within several years after transplantation. Factors that predispose to this complication include older age, black race, and obesity. With the exceptions of MMF and azathioprine, most immunosuppressive medications used in transplantation have been noted to be diabetogenic; glucocorticoids and tacrolimus especially predispose patients to PTDM. Screening for PTDM should be a routine part of post-transplant care. The pathophysiology of this condition is similar to that of type 2 diabetes, and it involves impaired insulin resistance and impaired insulin secretion. PTDM should be treated as aggressively as other forms of diabetes. Therapy should include lifestyle modifications as well as oral agents and insulin. Patients with PTDM should be screened

for all complications of diabetes, including diabetic nephropathy as per established diabetes care standards.

Cancer

(J Am Soc Nephrol 2004;15:1582)
Surveillance for malignant conditions is an important aspect of the long-term care of kidney transplant recipients. Several factors predispose transplant recipients to cancer. These include immunosuppression, conventional risk factors such as age and smoking, infections with viruses such as hepatitis B and C, human papillomavirus, and HHV 8. Prior to transplantation and ESRD, patients may have a history of treatment with cyclophosphamide for autoimmune disease or cancer. Cyclophosphamide itself is a risk factor for transitional cell carcinoma. Substantial geographic variations in the epidemiology of post-transplant malignancy exist. Liver cancer is common in Asia, where viral hepatitis is common. In Japan, where gi cancers are more common than in other countries, they also constitute the most common malignancy after transplantation. In Queensland, Australia, where a Caucasian population resides in an environment with a high level of sun exposure, the incidence of skin cancer rises from 7% 1 year after transplant to nearly 70% 20 years after the transplant (Transplantation 1996;61:715).

Malignancy may arise de novo in a transplant recipient after transplantation. It can also be present prior to transplantation or be transmitted with a graft. Some types of cancer are substantially more common in kidney transplant patients than in the general population. This problem is especially important in the patients who have functioning transplants for over 10 yr. In these patients, the risk of developing cancer is more than 10 times higher than in the general population and than in those patients who remain on dialysis because of the inability to receive a kidney transplant (Lancet 1999;354:93). Not all cancers present with the same level of increased risk. The 2 most common malignancies after transplantation are the PTLD occurring during the first post-transplant year, and squamous cell carcinomas of the skin and female genital organs. The ratio of the risk of some cancers observed in kidney transplant recipients vs expected in the general population at 5 to 9 yr after transplantation is as follows (Int J Cancer 1995;60:183):

- Skin cancer – 18
- Kidneys, ureters, bladder – 8
- Lymphoma – 7
- Lungs and respiratory system – 5
- Gastrointestinal system – 3

Given the dramatic increase in cancer risk shown above, cancer screening is important in this patient population. Skin cancer prevention and screening are critical. All transplant recipients should be educated about sun avoidance, use of protective clothing, and correct use of sunscreen. Expert panels recommend annual or more frequent, when necessary, skin examinations by a dermatologist. Practice guidelines are available on this topic (Nephrol Dial Transplant 2002;17[suppl 4]:31). Annual screening for female gynecological cancers is also recommended, along with appropriate screening for colorectal cancer. In addition, some experts recommend routine annual screening for urinary system cancers with screening for hematuria as well as annual imaging of the kidneys with ultrasound or CT (J Am Soc Nephrol 2000;11[suppl 15]:S1).

Index

transplant candidates and, 306
Antiphospholipid antibody syndrome, 138, 145
Antipsychotics, catecholamine levels, 291t
Anti-Il2 receptor antibodies, 315
APLAs. See Antiphospholipid antibodies
Apparent resistant hypertension, 277
Aquaporins, 8, 24
ARB-induced prerenal azotemia. See ACEI- and ARB-induced prerenal azotemia
ARBs. See Angiotensin-receptor blockers
ARPKD. See Autosomal recessive polycystic kidney disease
Arteriovenous fistula complications, 226–33
Arteriovenous fistulas, 222
    creating, 218–19
    infections in, 229–31
    KDOQI thrombosis and patency goals for, 227t
    rates, 221
    at the wrist, 219
Arteriovenous grafts, 218
    aneurysms in, 231–32
    creating, 219–20
    infections in, 229–31
    KDOQI thrombosis and patency goals for, 227t
    thrombosis and, 222
    vascular steal syndrome and, 232–33, 232t
Aspirin ingestion, salicylate poisoning and, 41–42
Asthma, 52
Asymptomatic gross hematuria, 113–14
Asymptomatic microscopic hematuria, 112–13
Asymptomatic non-nephrotic proteinuria, 115
Atherosclerotic disease, of renal arteries, 285
ATN. See Acute tubular necrosis
Atrial natriuretic peptide, 267
Atropine, 292
Auscultatory method, of blood pressure measurement, 272
Australia, skin cancer and kidney transplant recipients in, 340
Autoimmune diseases
    secondary membranoproliferative glomerulonephritis and, 139
    Type 1 (distal) renal tubular acidosis and, 45t
Autoimmune (idiopathic) TTP, 100
Autologous stem cell transplant, AL amyloidosis and, 154
Automated blood pressure devices, 271

Autosomal dominant Alport syndrome, 159
Autosomal dominant polycystic kidney disease, 163–65
Autosomal recessive Alport syndrome, 159
Autosomal recessive polycystic kidney disease, 165–66
AVFs. See Arteriovenous fistulas
AVGs. See Arteriovenous grafts
Azathioprine, 146, 321, 333, 339
Azotemia, 56, 73, 74
    prerenal, 61–64

B

Banff classification, acute rejection typing and, 325
Bartter's syndrome, 10, 15, 48, 180
Basement membrane thickness
    controversy over normal range of, 161–62
    light chain deposition disease and, 150
Basiliximab, 315
B blood group, kidney transplantation and, 296
B cell disorders, 137
B cell lymphoma, 149, 152
Bence-Jones proteinuria, 110
Benign familial hematuria, 158
Benign orthostatic proteinuria, 114
    epidemiology, 114
    laboratory screening, 114
Beta blockers, 18t, 291
    hypertensive patients and, 269, 270
ß-thalassemia, 166
Bisphosphonates, 25, 337
    multiple myeloma-associated acute kidney injury and, 96
BK polyomavirus nephropathy, 331–34
Blacks. See African Americans
Blindness, irreversible, methanol ingestion and, 40
Blood flow, through dialyzer, 214
Blood groups, kidney transplantations and, 296
Blood pressure
    JNC 7 classification, 267t
    normal, criteria for, 272t
Blood pressure control
    in different settings, 272t
    proteinuria and, 123
Blood pressure cuff sizes, recommended, 273t
Blood pressure measurement, 271–74
Bone and mineral metabolism in ESRD and CKD, 197–204
Bone density measurement, persistent post-transplant hyperparathyroidism and, 337

diabetic nephropathy and, 120
dialysis catheter complications, 233–39
epidemiology of, in U.S., 205–10, 205t
heavy chain deposition disease and, 151
hemodialysis access, 217–22
hemodialysis adequacy, 222–26
hemodialysis principles and prescription, 210–17
IgA nephropathy and, 141
incidence of, in U.S., 207
light chain deposition disease and, 150
mortality in patients with, 208
number of patients with, in U.S., 206
nutritional issues and, 260–63
peritoneal dialysis, 240
peritoneal dialysis adequacy, 244–48
peritoneal dialysis complications, 248–60
peritoneal dialysis principles and prescription, 240–44
prevalence of, in U.S., 208, 208
systemic lupus erythematosus nephritis and, 144
Enteric-coated mycophenolate sodium, 322
Enteric hyperoxaluria, 179
Epinephrine, 266
Eplerenone, 18t, 51
Eprodisate, 155
Epstein-Barr virus, post-transplantation lymphoproliferative disorders and, 334
Erythrocytosis, post-transplant, 335–36
Erythropoietic stimulating agents, 195–96
Erythropoietin, 193, 336
Erythropoietin alpha, 195
Erythropoietin deficiency, chronic kidney disease and, 192
ESAs. See Erythropoietic stimulating agents
Esmolol, 280
Ethacrinic acid, 28
Ethanol, 40
Ethnicity, end stage renal disease and, 206–7, 207
Ethylene glycol levels, determination of, 32
Ethylene glycol poisoning, 39–41
Euvolemic, hypoosmolar hyponatremia, 1
Exit site care, peritoneal dialysis peritonitis and, 251
Exit site infections, 233, 254

F

Fabrazyme, 168
Fabry disease, 167–68
Factor V Leiden, 306
Factor V Leiden mutations, 226, 227
Familial Mediterranean fever, 154

Fanconi syndrome, 46
Febuxostat therapy, 182
Females. See also Women
    Alport syndrome and, 159
    reflux nephropathy and, 172
Fenoldopam nicardipine, 280
Fentanyl, 292
Ferritin, 194, 196
Fibrillary glomerulonephritis, 138, 156
Fistula First initiative, 221
Fistula rates, in U.S., 221
Fistulograms, 228, 229
5-oxoproline, 37
Fludrocortisone, AL amyloidosis and, 154
Flumazenil, 52
Focal segmental glomerulosclerosis, primary, 126–29
Foley catheter
    abdominal compartment syndrome and, 90
    bladder obstruction and, 107
Folic acid, 41
Fomepizole, 40
Fourth National Health and Nutrition Examination Survey, 192–93
Fractional excretion of sodium, 69
    calculating, 63
Fractional excretion of urea, calculating, 63
Freely filtered light chains, 95
Free water deficit, calculating, 8
FSGS. See Focal segmental glomerulosclerosis
Fungal infections, peritoneal dialysis and, 253
Furosemide, 25, 28

G

Gadolinium
    hypocalcemia and, 20
    nephrogenic skin sclerosis and, 286
Galactosemia, Type 2 (proximal) renal tubular acidosis and, 45t
Gallium nitrate, 25
Ganciclovir, 331
Gastrointestinal potassium loss, 11
Gender. See also Females; Males; Men; Women
    AL amyloidosis and, 152
    Alport syndrome and, 158
    end stage renal disease and, 206–7
    fibrillary glomerulonephritis and, 156
    hypertension and, 266
    hypertensive crises and, 279
    IgA nephropathy and, 140
    reflux nephropathy and, 172
    systemic lupus erythematosus and, 143

S

Salicylate level, laboratory tests for, 32
Salicylate poisoning, 41–42
Sandimmune, 317
SBP. *See* Spontaneous bacterial peritonitis
Schistosomiasis, 305
Scleroderma renal damage, 138
Sclerosing peritonitis, 255–56
SCUF. *See* Slow continuous ultrafiltration
Secondary aldosteronism, 288
Secondary amyloidosis, 154–55
Secondary chronic interstitial nephritis, 169
Secondary focal segmental
  glomerulosclerosis, 128, 130–31
  hypertension and, 118
Secondary hypertension, 265, 277
Secondary IgA nephropathy, 139, 140
Secondary membranoproliferative
  glomerulonephritis, 136–39
Secondary nephrotic syndrome, 116t
Second National Health and Nutrition
  Examination Survey, 190
Self-Measurement of Blood Pressure at Home
  in the Elderly: Assessment and Follow-up
  study, on masked hypertension, 276
Sepsis, 57
Septic abortion, ATN due to, 103
Serum albumin, measuring, for dialysis
  patients, 261
Serum bicarbonate, abnormal, acid-base
  disorder and, 31
Serum calcium, reducing, 25
Serum creatinine, diabetic nephropathy
  and, 123
Serum potassium levels, complications with,
  14
Serum potassium test, hypertension and, 268
Sevelamer carbonate, 202
Sevelamer hydrochloride, 201
Seventh Report of the Joint National
  Committee on Prevention, Detection,
  Evaluation and Treatment of High Blood
  Pressure, 265
Severe pre-eclampsia
  complications, 282
  defined, 281
SHEAF study. *See* Self-Measurement of
  Blood Pressure at Home in the Elderly:
  Assessment and Follow-up study
Sheehan's syndrome, 8
Shell vial method, rapid CMV culture by, 330
SIADH, 1
Sickle cell nephropathy, 138, 166–67
Simulect, 315

Sirolimus, 320–21, 328
  drug interactions, 318t, 321
Sjögren's syndrome, Type 1 (distal) renal
  tubular acidosis and, 44, 45t
Skeletal system, chronic kidney disease and,
  197–98
Skin cancer
  kidney transplantation and, 308
  kidney transplant recipients and, 340, 341
SLE. *See* Systemic lupus erythematosus
SLEDD. *See* Slow low efficiency daily dialysis
Sleep apnea, 51, 52
  resistant hypertension and, 277–78
Slow continuous ultrafiltration, 59–60
Slow low efficiency daily dialysis, 61
Smoking
  diabetic nephropathy and, 124
  hypertension and, 266
Sodium excess, total body, 27–29
Sodium polystyrene (kayexalate), 97–98
Sodium polystyrene sulfonate, 19
Sodium restriction, 28
Soft tissues, chronic kidney disease and,
  198–99
Sotalol, 291
"Spikes" in capillary wall, membranous
  nephropathy and, 133
Spironolactone, 18t, 29, 51
Spontaneous bacterial peritonitis,
  hepatorenal syndrome and, 93
Spot albumin to creatinine ratio, 122
Squamous cell carcinomas, kidney transplant
  recipients and, 341
Staphylococcus aureus infection, 231
  catheter sepsis and, 234, 235
  exit site infections and, 254
  peritoneal dialysate leaks and, 260
  treating, 252
Starvation ketoacidosis, 39
Statins, post-transplant dyslipidemia and,
  339
Stenosis, access recirculation and, 224, 225
Stenosis in AVF and AVG, 226–29
Steroids
  focal segmental glomerulosclerosis and, 128
  IgA nephropathy and, 142–43
  light chain deposition disease and, 150
  membranous nephropathy and, 133
  minimal change disease and, 124, 125
"Stone clinic effect," 178
Strongyloides, 305
Struvite stone disease, 183–84
Studies of Left Ventricular Dysfunction
  (SOLVD trial), 64